P9-ARL-492

The Diabetic and the Dietitian

How to Help Your Husband Defeat Diabetes… without Losing Your Mind or Marriage!

WITHDRAWN

Also by Ellen and Michael Albertson

*Food as Foreplay: Recipes for
Romance, Love and Lust*

*Temptations: Igniting the Pleasure
and Power of Aphrodisiacs*

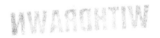
WITHDRAWN

The Diabetic and the Dietitian

How to Help Your Husband Defeat Diabetes... without Losing Your Mind or Marriage!

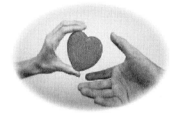

Dr. Ellen Albertson, PhD, MS, RDN, CD
Michael Albertson, Recovering Diabetic

ALEXANDRIA PRESS
Burlington, Vermont

The Diabetic and the Dietitian: How to Help Your Husband Defeat Diabetes... without Losing Your Mind or Marriage
Copyright © 2016 by Michael and Ellen Albertson

All Rights Reserved, including the right of reproduction in whole or in part in any form. No part of this publication can be reproduced, stored in a retrieval system, or transmitted in any form or by any means, electronic, mechanical, photocopying, recording, scanning, methods yet invented or otherwise, except as permitted under sections 107 or 108 of the 1976 United States Copyright Act, without prior written permission of the Publisher. Request to the Publisher for permission should be addressed to: Permissions, Alexandria Press, P.O. Box 5355, Burlington, VT 05404.

First Printing
Printed in the United States of America
10 9 8 7 6 5 4 3 2

All calorie and carbohydrate estimates and nutrition information is from the United States Department of Agriculture National Nutrient Database for Standard Reference and the Academy of Nutrition and Dietetics.

This book presents the experiences, opinions and ideas of the authors concerning the subject areas addressed herein. It is intended to provide helpful and informative material. It is sold with the understanding that the authors and publisher are not engaged in rendering medical, health, or any other kind of personal professional services in the book. It is not intended to substitute for personal consultations with health care professionals. The reader should consult his or her medical, health, or other competent professional before adopting any of the suggestions in this book or drawing inferences from it.

The authors and publisher specifically disclaim all responsibility for any liability, loss, or risk, personal or otherwise, which is incurred as a consequence, directly or indirectly, of the use and application of any of the contents of this book.

Editor: Jon Ford
Cover and interior designed by Joyce Weston

Contents

If your husband has type 2 diabetes or is prediabetic, you can't live without this book!
—Neither can he.

Introduction

You've just received the news: your husband has been diagnosed with prediabetes or type 2 diabetes. Or maybe he already has diabetes and has been ignoring it. Either way, you're worried about him and your future together . . . and rightfully so. Diabetes is the seventh leading cause of death in the United States. If left untreated, diabetes can cause kidney failure, nerve damage, heart disease, gum disease, erectile dysfunction, blindness, and depression.

Suddenly the dream of a long, loving life and happy retirement together filled with traveling and visits from grandkids is fading to black. Nagging, begging, bribing, and hiding the chips haven't worked. You feel isolated and alone. Not sure what to do or where to turn for trustworthy information and support. His doctor (who he ignores) is there for him, but who's helping you?

Hi, I'm Michael, the diabetic. My wife, Ellen, is the dietitian. She's also a food psychologist and all-around great human being who helped me defeat diabetes. When I was diagnosed with type 2 diabetes, we discovered that there were no books or reference materials available to specifically help wives deal with and help their husbands defeat this common condition. We wrote this book together to help you!

Type 1 Diabetes

Type 1 diabetes is an autoimmune disorder in which the body attacks the cells in the pancreas that make insulin. Type 1 diabetes, previously known as juvenile diabetes, has no cure, but it can be managed. People with the disease *must* take insulin for their entire lives to function properly and prevent life-threatening tissue damage.

This book does not address type 1 diabetes. If your husband has type 1 diabetes, he should consult his doctor to determine the best treatment options.

We know his diabetes is affecting the whole family . . . especially you. We are here to support you and provide expert advice to help your man in easy, simple-to-understand language. This book is designed to provide the psychological support you need, something all those MD-written diabetic books never address. Reading those jargon-filled medical texts, you'd think that wives don't exist. Well, you do exist, and you are the key to your husband's recovery. Not his doctor . . . you! His doctor can't reverse diabetes, but believe it or not, you can . . . and we're going to show you exactly how. Ellen did it for me, and we can help you do it with your husband too!

According to the Centers for Disease Control and Prevention (CDC), 15.5 million, or 13.6 percent, of American men have diabetes. Another 86 million American adults are estimated to have prediabetes, a condition that if left untreated will progress into full-blown diabetes. There are millions of women just like you facing the diabetic dilemma: How do I help my husband get healthy without losing my mind or my marriage?

Dollars and Diabetes

In 2012, diabetes and its related complications accounted for $245 billion in total medical costs and lost work and wages. This figure is up from $174 billion in 2007. The Centers for Disease Control and Prevention estimates that as many as one-third of adults in the United States will have diabetes by 2050! (But not if we can help it.)

No one needs another 400-page book discussing the scientific details of diabetes. Wives need a guide, written in clear, nonmedical English, that the average person can understand, with actionable information and guidelines they can use to help their husbands defeat diabetes and regain optimum health. Yes, ladies, your partner can defeat diabetes . . . just like I did. But he's going to need your help to take control of his health and maintain a long, healthy life. I would not have defeated diabetes without the love and support of my amazing wife and the life-saving strategies she designed and implemented for me. Not only do I feel better and have more energy than I've had in years, defeating diabetes is a shared victory that strengthened our marriage and brought us closer together.

I know what you're thinking: "Of course he could do it. He's married to a medical professional." True. And that's one of the reasons why we wrote this book—to share the nutrition science and psychological strategies Ellen developed to bring my A1C (a test that measures blood sugar average over a three-month period) down from 7.8 to 6.3 in less than a year. I lost 25 pounds and lowered my blood glucose levels naturally, without toxic medications or insulin. I am now diabetes-free . . . and will stay that way by using the amazingly effective psychological techniques and dietary strategies we are about to share with you.

The Diabetic and the Dietitian is very different than any other medical book you have ever read . . . or, for that matter, any other medical book that's ever been published. That's because in this book you will get the wife's perspective (Ellen), the husband's perspective (me), and at times our combined voice as we walk you through the diabetic journey from diagnosis to recovery to finally defeating diabetes and maintaining a healthy, energetic, diabetes-free existence for the rest of your partner's life.

Unlike typical diabetes books, which only cover diet and exercise, we address the nutrition and lifestyle changes he needs to make AND we provide proven psychological techniques you can use to help him make and maintain those changes . . . for the rest of his life.

We provide the nutrition tools, psychological strategies and insights, easy-to-follow food guidelines, and critical support you both need. Most important, you'll gain the confidence and knowledge to help him defeat diabetes starting today . . . even if he doesn't want to change his lifestyle at all. (That's why Ellen is going to teach you those psychological techniques. ☺)

As a matter of fact, Ellen would like to make a couple of points now . . .

The lion's share of diabetic books are written by ivory tower academic researchers or wealthy, skinny, Madison Avenue diet docs. But here's the problem: most of these people haven't struggled with diabetes themselves. They might know the science, but they don't know and understand the emotions, challenges, depressions, and impact that diabetes has on regular families with normal, North American lifestyles.

We understand what you and your husband are going through because we've lived it . . . and beat it. And beating diabetes is not as hard as you think. Plus, unlike registered dietitians and psychologists, MDs receive very little (if any) nutritional and psychological instruction in medical school. They just aren't trained to effectively help people eat right and permanently change their behavior. (But it does seem like a lot of them took an advanced course in talking-too-fast, doesn't it?)

As a PhD psychologist, registered dietitian, licensed nutritionist, and certified wellness coach who's worked with thousands of people just like you, I've made sure to provide you with the latest information to help your husband live well with, control, and reverse diabetes. This book is a comprehensive guide that contains only factual, actionable, medical information and powerful techniques and recommendations to get your husband healthy ASAP. And you won't lose your mind or marriage in the process.

I've read all the medical texts (pretty boring) and have compiled all the relevant information you'll need here in this book so you don't have to spend days online or at the library figuring out what to do and how to do it. I've done it all and tested it on my own husband so you don't have to. Everything you need to defeat diabetes is in your hands right now.

This book is written for the partner of a diabetic because in reality, let's face it, ladies, we keep the family healthy and do most of the food shopping, cooking, and cleanup. (According to a Labor Department survey, on an average day, women do more than 2 times the amount of food preparation and cleanup as men do.) Whether this is good or bad, fair or unfair, feminist or regressive, doesn't matter. This book is not political. All Michael and I are interested in is helping you get him, and keep him, healthy again.

This book will not only help you understand what diabetes is; more importantly, through Michael's experience, we will explain what your husband is going through emotionally due to his diagnosis. Men don't usually talk about these things, even to their wives. So, Michael has invaluable insights and advice to share about how men react emotionally and how you can channel these emotions in a positive way to turn diabetic depression into motivation to live a full, fantastic, diabetes-free life.

In addition to showing you how to keep hubby healthy, we're going to teach you life-changing psychological coping techniques so he doesn't drive you crazy as you save his health. I know it can be a pain, ladies, but if we don't take care of these beasts, who will?

"That was kind of a cheap shot, Ellen."
"Quiet, Michael, this is woman talk."

As I was saying . . . you and I will discuss his conflicting emotions and the psychologically fragile state a diabetic diagnosis creates in most men, as well as how to deal with it while protecting your own emotional health . . . without Michael interrupting.

Now here's the big secret we don't want to tell the boys. By working together to reverse his diabetes, you're going to lose weight, feel great, and boost your own health too! Commit to our easy program and you'll both feel better than you have in years.

Diabetes is a wake-up call. If he doesn't answer it, his future—to put it politely—is grim. But by reading this book, you have taken the first important step on his road to recovery. Now, let me turn it back over to Michael . . .

Diabetes is sneaky. Even though I was exercising and my diet was relatively healthy (I'm married to a dietitian, after all), the natural biological changes that occur with aging make it easy for diabetes to slither into your system. It just takes an extra pound or two per year and suddenly you're 20, 30, 40 pounds overweight. The doc is talking about blood sugar, insulin, needles and threatening that if you don't take a bunch of powerful drugs with negative side effects you could get kidney damage, cataracts, glaucoma, heart disease, stroke, nerve damage, and foot problems that could lead to amputations . . .

Amputations? What the . . .

Just like I did, your husband probably watched doc's mouth move in disbelief. One scary fact after another poured out as hubby thought to himself, "What is he talking about? Diabetes? Me? No way. I'm just a little overweight. I lift weights, shoot hoops with the guys, and eat broccoli, low-fat potato chips, and only drink beer on game days. (Okay, you can always find a game on ESPN, but still!) Doc must have gotten my blood test mixed up with some 400-pound coach potato watching *Law and Order* reruns all day."

As I drove home the day I got my diagnosis, I was upset, confused, and thinking . . . my life is over. I'm getting . . . no, I am old. No more fun, all my favorite foods . . . gone. Rabbit grub and cardboard cuisine forever. How did this happen? Will I have to inject myself? Prick myself multiple times per day to monitor my blood sugar? Will I lose my eyesight or need to go on dialysis from kidney damage? Taking care of diabetes is expensive. How are we going to pay the medical bills? How many years is diabetes going to take from my life? Will I ever be able to eat cheesecake again? What did I do to deserve this?

It's hard for all of us diabetic men to accept, not just your mate.

But you both need to understand—diabetes is not the end; it's just a new challenge that, with a little creativity and determination, can be defeated without resorting to expensive medications, draconian diets, or soul-crushing workouts. He's still going to get tasty, fun, filling food. In fact, continuing to eat the foods he loves while introducing new, healthier options is a key element in reversing diabetes. (Ellen will teach you how to infiltrate healthy foods into his diet without him noticing in chapters 8 and 12.) He can still have beer, wine, or a cocktail, and you're going to help him adjust his diet to accommodate these calories.

You don't have to let diabetes leach the fun out of life. The transition the two of you are going through (yes, it's a transition . . . and a challenge for both of you) doesn't mean the end of fun or good food. You can still have a long, loving, fun life together filled with vitality and romance. You two can and will travel, eat out, and enjoy life. We're going to show you how.

The beauty of diabetes (if one can say there is beauty in a disease) is he really can heal himself . . . and it's not that hard! With several dietary tweaks, a little exercise, and some mindful eating (more on mindful eating in chapter 4), you and your husband, working together, will defeat diabetes. We did! And just as Ellen promised, it was easier than I thought.

His diabetes diagnosis isn't a death sentence. In fact, this diagnosis just saved his life.

Let's get started on saving that life—and helping you cope with the changes he's going through—right now!

Chapter 1

Diabetes, In Plain English
Understanding the Problem

Diabetes is a disease that occurs when the body cannot properly control blood sugar (also called glucose) levels. When someone has diabetes, his blood sugar levels rise above the normal, healthy range. While glucose is vital to health (it's an important energy source for cells, tissues, and organs and the main source of fuel for the brain), high blood sugar is bad for your body and can lead to serious complications. That's why it's so important to keep his blood sugar levels as normal as possible.

Glucose vs. Sugar: What's the Difference?

In this book we use the terms "blood glucose" and "blood sugar" interchangeably. They mean the exact same thing: The sugar that is transported through the bloodstream to supply energy to all the body's cells.

There are three types of diabetes. In addition to type 1 mentioned in the introduction and type 2, which is what this book is about, there's one more type of diabetes: gestational. Gestational diabetes occurs during pregnancy and so obviously isn't an issue for your man.

The human body likes balance, which is why it normally keeps blood sugar levels within a fairly narrow range. To maintain consistent blood sugar levels, an organ called the pancreas (which sits behind your stomach) secretes two hormones: insulin and glucagon.

"Glucagon? I think I saw those guys in concert once."
"Michael. This isn't a comedy club. Stop heckling me."

"This is pretty heavy stuff. I was just trying to lighten the mood."
"Can you lighten the mood without interrupting me?"
"But that wouldn't be any fun."
"This isn't fun . . . it's science!"
"I love it when you get angry about science. It's very sexy."

Did I mention that one of the benefits of defeating diabetes is increased libido . . . on *his* part? You've been warned.

Normally, when blood sugar gets too high the pancreas releases insulin, which allows blood sugar to either enter cells so it can be used for energy or stored as fat. If blood sugar gets too low the pancreas secretes glucagon, which signals the liver to release glycogen (a form of stored glucose) into the bloodstream so blood sugar levels rise.

When someone has type 2 diabetes, insulin isn't working correctly. As a result, instead of being used for energy, sugar piles up in the bloodstream, driving glucose levels higher and higher. The body secretes more and more insulin to lower blood sugar levels, but the cells resist using the insulin. Eventually this insulin resistance can get so bad his body can't make enough insulin to control blood sugar levels.

Then, the dangerous diabetic cycle kicks in: That extra blood sugar gets stored as fat and weight increases, which makes blood sugar shoot up even higher! The pancreas starts to wear out and as a result can't produce enough insulin. That's when type 2 diabetics MUST start injecting insulin to reduce blood sugar levels. (Follow the recommendations in this book and your husband can avoid the insulin needle . . . forever.)

Meanwhile, as his blood sugar levels rise his energy plummets, because his cells are literally starved for fuel. He feels tired and, because his energy is so low, he's driven by food cravings. This dynamic makes it really tough to exercise and eat right and almost impossible to lower blood sugar! Since the brain operates entirely on glucose, those high blood sugar levels impact his mood and thinking. He may have trouble concentrating and become a very grumpy camper. Sound like anyone you know?

While genes play a role in the development of type 2 diabetes, it's environmental factors such as poor eating habits and a sedentary lifestyle that trigger the disease. Studies show that high body mass index (BMI), excess belly fat (visceral fat), low intake of fiber, and physical inactivity are all associated with an increased risk of developing type 2 diabetes. To put it simply: they weigh too much, eat too much, and move too little . . . in other words, most American men over 35.

Now for the good news: type 2 diabetes is reversible!

Research Shows Diabetes is Reversible

A study conducted at Newcastle University and published in the scientific journal *Diabetologia* found that when individuals restricted calories, they started making enough insulin AND their cells responded to it normally. Another study of over 5,000 overweight adults conducted at the University of Alabama at Birmingham and published in the *Journal of the American Medical Association* (JAMA) found that lifestyle interventions, including diet and exercise, can put type 2 diabetes into remission and eliminate the need for medication.

It's true! There is a natural, drug-free solution for diabetes and prediabetes that's safer, nontoxic, works better, and is cheaper than all those high-priced, side effect–laden, toxic medications. Research conducted by the Diabetes Prevention Program, a landmark clinical study that followed a group of diabetics for 10 years, found medication did not work nearly as well as lifestyle change to control the disease.

Many medications actually make diabetes worse by pushing the pancreas to produce more insulin, which wears it out faster. Common side effects of some diabetes medications include weight gain, nausea, vomiting, and liver damage. Some medications, such as a class of drugs called sulfonylureas, are so dangerous the US Food and Drug Administration (FDA) requires a special black box warning stating that these drugs can increase the risk of a heart attack! Other medications are so new that the dangers have yet to be revealed.

No matter how long he's struggled in vain against type 2 diabetes, he now has a real opportunity to defeat diabetes and achieve trouble-free blood sugar—quickly. Losing just 5 to 10 percent of his body weight will improve his blood sugar levels. If he's prediabetic (in other words, his blood sugar level is higher than normal, but it's not yet high enough to be classified as type 2 diabetes), losing 5 to 10 percent of his body weight will lower his risk of developing diabetes by 58 percent! Without intervention, prediabetes will almost surely progress to type 2 diabetes, resulting in debilitating and life-threatening damage to his body.

Fortunately, the progression from prediabetes to diabetes to serious medical complications and reduced life expectancy isn't inevitable. Regardless of his age and stage of diabetes, view his diagnoses as an opportunity to save his health starting right NOW. You can help him bring his blood sugar level back to normal and reverse diabetes and its complications by following the simple, straightforward program in this book!

Let's start with . . .

SET, POINT . . . MATCH!

Everyone has a "set point," i.e., the body weight they normally fluctuate around, which is determined by genes and environment. The secret to lowering his set point—and this is one of the keys to defeating diabetes—is working *with*, not against, the body.

Humans evolved when food was scarce (there just weren't that many Jiffy Marts around during the Stone Age), so we're designed to maintain, not lose weight. That's great when you're starving to death and praying that Atouk kills a mammoth . . . soon! Not so great for a diabetic-vulnerable America in the twenty-first century.

Even though the cupboard is full and there's a 24/7 McDonald's around the corner, when you lose weight too quickly your body still thinks it's 15,000 BC and you're starving to death. To maintain life when you're calorie deprived, the body releases hormones that rev up appetite and fat storage and reduce metabolism so you slow down and burn fewer calories. The result is you feel hungry, agitated, and tired and can't stop thinking about food! Which, needless to say, makes it impossible to lose weight and keep it off. Conversely, when weight is lost slowly and steadily by eating a healthy, nutrient-rich diet, the body feels great and adjusts to the lower set point without going into starvation mode.

THE RESET EQUATION

Now let's talk about resetting *his* set point. To start, the two of you set an initial goal of losing 10 percent of his weight over a specific period of time. For example, if he weighs 250 pounds, shoot for losing 25 pounds initially over 6 months. That's about a pound per week, easily doable. Here's how, in two simple steps:

1. Cut back his daily calories by 15–20 percent, about 300–500 calories per day. That's as easy as skipping one order of fries (330 calories), two sodas (300 calories), or a candy bar (350 calories), or ordering plain coffee instead of a Chocolate Chip Coolatta (800 calories) at Dunkin' Donuts.
2. Help him commit to one or two of these changes per week.

Really, that's it. Follow those two steps and the weight will effortlessly come off, without his body fighting back. That's the beauty of our program—no diets, no drastic food reduction, and no starvation strategies. Just slow, steady, EASY changes.

News flash: men tend to be competitive. He'll probably think, "I can lose more than that." Your job is to remind him that this is a marathon, not a sprint. A slow, gradual approach that resets his set point will help prevent what we call *hanger* (hunger + anger = *hanger*) and instead leave him *happyfied* (happy + satisfied = *happyfied*).

When he loses the first 10 percent of excess weight, hold at that point and work on maintaining the loss. He's reached goal number one. Let him celebrate a little. (Emphasis on a *little,* please. No weeklong pizza and beer binges.) After a few days, remind him that if he's lost 10 percent he can lose another 10. Then, go for the next 10 percent. Continue this pattern until he reaches a healthy, diabetes-free weight. (Don't worry. We've mapped out the whole process for you in the coming chapters. Read on!)

As his body changes, tell him how fabulous he looks. Ask him how he feels. After just a 10 percent loss, he should feel noticeably better. Diabetic symptoms like foot pain, sluggishness, erectile dysfunction, and brain fog will start to recede as his cells begin to process blood sugar again. That's right, just a 10 percent weight loss will make a big difference, a difference he *will* feel . . . and it *will* feel good—for *both* of you!

As you continue to get healthy together, it's important to be aware of several diabetic myths that might derail his progress. Let's look at those now . . .

DIABETIC MYTHS

There are a lot of myths, rumors, and disinformation about diabetes floating around out there. Friends and family might have already shared some of these so-called "facts" with you. We're going to tackle a few of the more common myths.

Diabetes Is a Death Sentence

No it's not! You and your partner have a tremendous amount of control over whether his diabetes or prediabetes worsens or improves. What he does starting today and going forward will have a major impact on his health. Trust us on this: helping him change his health habits will have a remarkable, swift, and noticeable effect. Diabetes is only a death sentence if you let it be.

Diabetes Isn't Really a Serious Disease

Yes it is! More people die from diabetic complications than breast cancer and AIDS combined, and two-thirds of people with diabetes die of heart disease or stroke. It doesn't have to be that way if you and your husband take positive action to defeat diabetes now!

Eating Too Much Sugar Causes Diabetes

Since type 2 diabetes means your body has trouble controlling blood sugar, it's easy to think that eating too much sugar causes diabetes. But it's not that simple. Diabetes is caused by a number of factors, including a family history of the disease and being overweight.

Although eating a lot of sugar can contribute to weight gain and other complications with diabetes, other foods that break down in the bloodstream quickly (such as white bread, pasta, or rice) can have an equally damaging impact. So while cutting down on sweets is important in reversing the disease (you can still eat sugar occasionally), it's not the only diet change he needs to make to get healthy. Cutting down on total calories from all sources (not just sweets) and increasing activity levels are both key to losing weight and reversing the disease.

You Can Catch Diabetes from Someone Else

No! Although researchers don't know all the reasons why people get diabetes, it's not contagious. You can't catch it like the flu. So yes, keep kissing your husband. Being affectionate is a great health move for both of you.

If You Have Diabetes You Can't Have Fun Anymore

Michael here, and let me tell you . . . that's BS. I'm having plenty of fun! And the two of you will too. Just watch, when he gets his diabetes under control his energy level will skyrocket! I felt like I knocked 15 years off . . . and started acting like it.

> "Actually, Michael started acting like he was 15 . . . years old!"
> "Got my mojo workin', baby."
> "Down, boy, down. Back to the book!"

People with Diabetes Must Eat Special Diabetic Foods

Not true. There's no need to buy "diabetic" or "dietetic" packaged foods that promise special advantages for diabetics. They are expensive, and some contain artificial sweeteners that can have a laxative effect, whether you want it or not. A healthy meal plan to defeat diabetes is the same healthy diet everyone should eat to maximize their wellness. Everything he needs is available at your local market. And in chapter 8 we're going to show you exactly what to buy and how to prepare healthy, delicious diabetes-defeating dinners. (Breakfast, lunch, and snacks too.)

If You Have Diabetes, You Can't Eat Starchy Foods Like Bread, Potatoes, or Pasta

Again, not true. While it's important to control the amount of carbohydrates you consume—and white bread, potatoes, and pasta are classic examples of high-carb foods—no specific foods are off limits. All your favorite foods, including starchy foods, can be enjoyed in moderation.

People with Diabetes Can't Eat Sweets or Chocolate

Another not true. Fact: sweets and chocolate are not "off limits" to people with diabetes. The key to sweets, just like carbs, is the amount one eats, not the food itself. Keep favorite fun foods on his menu. Allowing the occasional treat is the best way not to cheat!

Learning what diabetes *will do* to your husband is scary. But please remember, diabetes is not only treatable, it's EASILY REVERSABLE with simple diet and lifestyle changes. We go in depth on how to make this transition smoothly and tastily in the chapters ahead.

Chapter 2

He's Turning Into a Swinger! What Can I Do?
Surviving the Five Stages of Diabetic Grief (Both of You)

There's a lot of debate about how men deal with their feelings. As a man, let me say that we men deal with our feelings just fine ... by locking them up. But sometimes, for our health, we need to unlatch that box and let the feelings flow. This is especially so if your husband has been diagnosed with a potentially life-altering condition like diabetes.

Mood swings are extremely common in diabetics for several reasons. The brain is fueled entirely by blood sugar and requires a steady supply of it to function properly. Rapid changes in blood sugar levels (a common issue for diabetics) can have a major impact on mood. (Just think about how you feel when you're really hungry or have eaten too much.) Abnormally high and/or low blood sugar levels can make hubby feel grumpy, tired, nervous, or confused. Put simply, erratic blood sugar levels are bad for his brain.

The body and mind are connected, so his negative moods can also affect his blood sugar levels. Stressful emotions like frustration and anger trigger the release of a hormone called cortisol, which increases blood sugar, appetite, and the tendency to store fat around the middle. Then, elevated blood sugar levels make him feel even more frustrated and angry, which drives sugar levels even higher, creating an emotionally negative and health defeating feedback loop.

In addition, the fear, worry, and stress associated with managing diabetes can also generate their own set of negative mood swings, especially right after his initial diagnosis. There's a lot he needs to learn and change (most of us don't handle change well), which can leave him feeling angry, sad, overwhelmed, or depressed.

After being diagnosed with either diabetes or prediabetes, most men will enter a period of grieving. It might show as anger, depression, isolation, or other ways, but the source of this post-diagnosis shift in his psychological mood state is grief.

He is probably unaware that he is grieving. He might chalk it up to a "bad mood," "feeling a little blue," or being "under the weather." Most likely, he won't acknowledge that his "mood" is due to the diabetic diagnosis. But the fact is, he is grieving . . . for himself—his lost youth, diminished health, fear of the future, fear of losing lifelong pleasures like tasty food and sexual activity.

This type of grieving is natural when someone gets a diagnosis of a serious disease. It's a process he must pass through. But—and it's a big but—you can't let him settle into a permanent state of grief or allow diabetes to become a psychological swamp he wallows in. Feeling sorry for himself, blaming himself or others for his bad health or, worse, believing his situation is fate and there's nothing he can do—all of this leads to him giving up and not even trying to defeat diabetes . . . which is *very* defeatable at this stage.

He needs emotional support. Reassure him that you love him and find him attractive. He's still the same person; he just needs to get through this stage of the process so he . . . and you . . . can move on to a healthier, happier place.

THE FIVE STAGES OF DIABETIC GRIEF

The five stages of diabetic grief—denial, bargaining, anger, depression, and acceptance—are universal, normal, and experienced by people from all walks of life. Rich, poor, black, white, tall, short, or Oompa Loompas, diabetes doesn't care. This disease is an equal opportunity illness.

Your partner will spend different lengths of time working through each stage with alternating levels of intensity. He may not experience the stages in the order listed or go through them all, which is okay. While there are patterns to grieving, people experience a variety of different reactions. How he grieves will partially depend on his personality and temperament before he got diabetes, as well as how sudden the diagnosis was, i.e., did it come out of the blue, or has his doctor been warning him for years?

Don't push him through the process faster than he wants or is capable of. Accept that this is challenging and painful for him. Try and meet him where he is emotionally, not where you want him to be. Be patient, offer help, but DON'T become the diabetes police. Nagging him or trying to force him to change or "get over" the grief won't work and may make matters worse.

He needs to grieve. You need to make sure his grief leads to positive, healthy actions to defeat diabetes. Now let's take a look at each of the five stages of diabetic grief and how to deal with them.

Denial

Many people experience denial when they first learn they have diabetes. He's probably in denial if he has thoughts like:

> *"This isn't happening to me."*
> *"I don't eat that much."*
> *"I never eat sweets."*
> *"I'm only a little overweight."*
> *"They mixed my test up with someone else."*
> *"I lift weights twice a week. This can't be right!"*

Denial is a normal reaction when dealing with overwhelming emotions. It's a defense mechanism that buffers the immediate shock of the diagnosis. This stage may go on for as little as a day or as long as several weeks. Hopefully he will come to terms with the fact that he has diabetes and must learn how to deal with it.

If he doesn't, then you must accept the reality that *you* have to take action, because denial (i.e., believing he doesn't have diabetes or it's not serious) will lead to the negative health consequences we described earlier. You can't let that happen.

Here's what you can do to wake him from diabetic denial. First, educate yourself and gather information, which is exactly what you're doing by reading this book. Next, set a day and time to sit down with him and discuss the facts in a *loving, compassionate* way.

This is not the time for criticism and vague generalizations. Be specific, sincere, and speak from your heart.

During this conversation, it's important to use "I" statements. "I" statements take the focus away from him (after all, he probably just wants to retreat to his favorite refuge and pretend this isn't happening), and they don't come across as judgmental and accusatory as "you" statements might in these circumstances. For example, tell him right up front: "I love you and want you to be healthy and happy, but I'm very worried about you." Doesn't that sound better than "If *you* don't get control of this situation and lose some weight, *you* are going to die"?

Next, state the facts about diabetes, the bad and *especially* the good: "It's reversible. We can beat this. It won't be as hard as you think. I will help you."

If he stays in denial even after this loving approach, be patient and leave the door open. Don't give up. There's plenty you can still do. Bring healthier foods into the home and refuse to buy junk. If he wants Cheetos, he'll have to go buy them himself. Cook smaller, healthier meals. Take a daily walk and invite him to come with you. Identify other people who can support you. Enlist the rest of the family to adopt healthy lifestyle changes. If everyone is participating, it will be easier for him to adapt. After all, diabetic or not, none of us really *needs* another bowl of Fruit Loops.

Bargaining

"I'll exercise more if I can still have potato chips."
"I'll lose weight if you do too."
"I'll cut out pizza if I can still have ice cream."

Does any of this sound familiar? It may seem like him making excuses or trying to avoid what needs to be done, but your husband is actually trying to regain control to overcome feelings of helplessness and vulnerability by "negotiating" a better "deal." Soon he'll discover that diabetes doesn't negotiate . . . with anyone . . . ever.

Here are some tactics to help shift him from bargaining toward acceptance. Please note: these are not instantaneous solutions, because there aren't any. It might take some time for him to come to acceptance.

✓ *Don't offer him false hope or allow him to buy into false hope.* While there are practical things you can help him with such as eating better, don't support his desire to take the "science-shattering secret formula" **guaranteed** to cure diabetes that he saw advertised on a late-night infomercial, at $75 per bottle, not including shipping, handling, or other charges written in print too small to read that will be applied to your credit card without your approval.

✓ *Resist the urge to set him straight.* For example, don't chastise him for gaining 35 pounds. That will just create defensiveness and hostility. This is not the time to remind him of his daily affair with Ben & Jerry's ice cream or his Saturday night pepperoni pizza habit that also falls on Tuesdays and Thursdays.

✓ *Don't defend his doctor.* This is a subcategory of setting him straight. You may be tempted to say something like, "Why won't you listen to Dr. Smarts? He knows more about this than you do." (Notice the accusatory "you" statements in there?) In your spouse's current agitated and confused state, that will just align you with the people he *thinks* are persecuting him.

✓ *Strike a win-win deal.* When men are in bargaining mode, sometimes there are things you can offer to motivate them to improve their health. Yes, we mean bribe him. Discuss a reward for meeting a health goal. For example, "If you lose 10 pounds you can buy that new _____" or "If you go to the gym three times per week for a month, I'll _____."

✓ *Humor him.* Listen to him. Smile and be understanding, even if you think what he's saying is silly, counterproductive, or pointless. You don't need to agree with him. But you do have to listen . . . sympathetically.

✓ *Make him feel valued and respected.* Doing so will help bolster him to accept rather than deny or bargain his way out of the situation. Show him you respect and believe in his judgment, abilities, and capabilities. Remind him that he's still the same guy you married. Diabetes hasn't changed that. But here's an important tip: avoid telling him how strong he is. For many men "strong" equals "silent," and silent equals bottling up his emotions.

Anger

Again, maybe you've already heard variations of the following:

"Jim down the street is bigger than me. Why doesn't he have diabetes?"

"Why didn't you make healthier meals?"

"What have I done to deserve this $#!&?" (Ladies, this is not the time to respond, *"Because you've been eating like a pig for years."*)

Reality and its pain merge. He's not ready to deal just yet. Give him space. He feels vulnerable and is redirecting painful emotions as anger, looking for an enemy. His anger and frustrations may initially be taken out on you, especially if you are the chief food service person in the home.

As much as you may want to, don't get angry in response. Remember, it's the grief talking.

But if you can't fight back, how *do* you survive this stage? Remember, you are not trying to fix him here (we start fixing him in chapter 3), or make the painful emotions disappear. You are just helping him deal with and move through these emotions in a productive way. Here are some ways to help him—and you—deal with his anger.

✓ *Don't react.* Stay calm. Let him talk and vent for as long as he likes. Respond with compassion and understanding—even if you don't feel like it.

✓ *Be loving.* Underneath all the bluster, he's confused and scared. Fear breeds anger. Responding with love will soothe and strengthen him. Instead of feeling alone and vulnerable, he'll feel respected, valued, and supported. This is how you begin the process of dissolving fear so he can eventually move to acceptance and action.

✓ *Reassure him.* Men perceive themselves as providers and protectors. That perception has been dented by diabetes. He's feeling vulnerable and insecure. He may be lashing out in an effort to feel powerful and in control. He's unlikely to acknowledge his doubts and fears at this point. Find ways to reassure him that he is the same man he's always been. The better he feels about himself, the better he will be able to defeat diabetes.

✓ *Don't take anything personally* (unless he starts throwing knives). It's the grief talking, not the person you love.

✓ *ASK what he needs* . . . since he probably won't tell you. If he says "I don't know" or "nothing," resist the urge to walk away frustrated or worried. Just keep being supportive however you can. Let him know you'll be there if he needs anything or would like to talk. He'll come around.

Depression

Depression comes when he wakes up from denial and/or realizes bargaining won't change the situation. You may hear things like:

"What's the point? There's nothing I can do."
"I guess this is what happens when you get old."
"I just can't deal with this."

It's very important to acknowledge and be aware that *diabetes and depression are linked.* Compared to people without the disease, diabetics have a greater risk of developing depression, and people with depression have a higher risk of developing diabetes—another dangerous health feedback loop.

The stress of managing diabetes, the negative effects it can have on the brain, and the extremes in blood sugar levels all contribute to depression. Depression may make him feel hopeless and decrease his desire and ability to embrace the lifestyle changes required to manage and defeat diabetes. Plus, many people overeat (especially high-calorie comfort foods) to self-soothe when they're depressed, which of course makes diabetes worse.

In most cases, mild depression is a natural part of the grieving process and will resolve itself without professional intervention. But if his depression lasts more than two weeks or is seriously interfering with his ability to interact with family or function at work, encourage him to talk to his doctor about getting properly diagnosed and treated by a mental health professional. Depression is an illness just like diabetes that requires special attention.

His Doctor and You

You need to make sure your husband goes to the doctor regularly and you need to take an active role in whatever medical advice he receives. Know what his medical instructions and care plan is. You may even want to visit the doctor with him if he's okay with that. Two heads and four ears are better than one when it comes to understanding what the doctor has to say, especially if your husband tends to get upset or emotional about medical matters. Men have a tendency to focus on the negative things doctors tell them. He might miss what he needs to do to improve his health. That's what you're there for. But . . . DO NOT approach his doctor without his permission. It's unethical and will undermine his faith and trust in you.

Don't be surprised if he doesn't want to take responsibility for his mental health. Not wanting to get treatment is often part of depression. If that is the case, enlist someone such as a family member, good friend, or anyone he respects who can support you on this. Agreeing to see a therapist is a big step for anyone, and frankly, he may need to hear it from someone besides just you.

But again, in most cases professional counseling will not be necessary, and there are plenty of other strategies you can use to lift him out of mild depression. Encourage him to be physically active and engage in activities (that *aren't* food oriented) that gave him pleasure prior to diabetes. Find ways to laugh and have fun. This will help remind him the world isn't ending and there's still plenty of enjoyment left. Yes, this is the time to rent some old Mel Brooks movies. (Michael recommends *Young Frankenstein*.) If you can, get away for a long weekend. A change of scenery often helps to change a mind.

Acceptance . . . and Action

Not everyone can reach this final stage on their own. *You* have to help him by being patient and supportive, just as you have been through the previous stages. Keep the faith. Eventually he will see that it is more painful and riskier to stay where he is than to take on the challenge of defeating diabetes. But first he has to accept the reality of the situation: *"I have diabetes. I have diabetes because of longstanding, unhealthy dietary habits. It's not going to go away unless I make it!"* Then, working together, the two of you develop his new *defeat diabetes action plan.*

How do you develop this plan? You don't have to—you're already holding it in your hand. This book IS his, and your, action plan. Now, use it!

In the next chapter, we're going to show you the first part of the plan—the most effective diabetic treatment known!

Chapter 3

The Most Effective Diabetic Treatment Known... Weight Loss

(Even If Men Don't Want to Admit It!)

"If you build it, he will come."
—*Field of Dreams*

"If you cook it, he will eat it."
—*Michael Albertson*

Ladies, you have more control over your husband's weight and helping him lower his set point than you realize. (Remember "set point" from chapter 1? It's the "normal" body weight—give or take a few pounds—for every individual.) When it comes to food, most of us men are pretty lazy—we'll eat what's presented to us. Is it sexist? Perhaps. Is it true? Yep. So this is where you get to use male laziness to help your man heal and defeat diabetes. Changing what you cook and serve him will have a *BIG* impact on his health, so this chapter is all about how to start leveraging that kitchen control.

And to the men who do cook, like me. Good for us! And don't tell the other guys about our secret: the quickest way to a woman's heart is to do the cooking. I can't tell you how many times I got . . .

"Michael, enough! We're supposed to be beating diabetes, not handing out romance tips. That was our first book."

"Oops, I didn't know you were listening, honey. Got carried away there for a minute, sorry. So let's move on to . . ."

After losing just a few pounds I was shocked—pleasantly so—at how I felt as glucose could finally get to my cells and do its job, providing energy and vitality. The pain in my feet that I thought was arthritis lessened, then vanished. Brain fog disappeared and libido reappeared. I started sleeping better, breathing easier, and experiencing less pain and inflammation throughout my body.

Your husband can feel the same relief and rejuvenation I did. We'll tell you exactly how in this chapter, but first, a little background on how differently men and women approach weight loss . . .

DIFFERENT STROKES FOR DIFFERENT FOLKS

You can't force him to lose weight, but you can help him help himself. To do so you have to understand how differently men and women think and feel about weight, weight loss, and dieting. There are specific physiological and psychological differences to how men and women approach weight loss. If you're going to help him defeat diabetes, you need to understand these differences.

Men generally will not talk about their feelings concerning weight. Men cope with feelings in other ways. (Generally by trying to ignore their feelings. It's the whole stoic, macho thing.) Which is why, now that he *has to lose weight or face dire health and mortality issues*, he needs your help.

As we discussed, for better or worse, women are generally more involved with grocery shopping and meal prep than most men. Which is where you come in. If you haven't already, you're going to have to take control of the food in your home. Yes, it is a bit sexist, but if you want him to defeat diabetes and have a healthy, vibrant, long life together . . . I'm sorry, but you really don't have a choice. My wonderful Michael is an exception. He shops, cleans, does laundry, *and* brings home the bacon. (I just don't let him eat too much of it!)

Fortunately, men tend to have an easier time losing weight than women. Speaking as a woman . . . that's annoying! But there's no arguing with biology so let's just move on.

MEN VS. WOMEN: TWO SIDES OF THE WEIGHT LOSS COIN

Men and women store and metabolize fat very differently. To ensure the survival of the species (it takes about 72,000 calories to grow a baby from conception to birth), women are designed to carry much more body fat than men. Women store this extra fat around the hips, butt, and legs. In contrast, men store fat around the belly, which is why they have beer bellies atop skinny legs.

Though the accumulation of lower body fat in women is harder to lose than male fat around the middle, it tends *not* to be a health issue. In fact, some research has shown that a little padding in the lower body is a sign of good health and fertility in women. (Take that, Kate Moss!) In contrast, the accumulation of abdominal fat in men (i.e., having a large waist circumference) is dangerous and strongly associated with inflammation, hypertension, insulin resistance, type 2 diabetes, and heart disease. Which means he's got to get rid of, or at least minimize, the waste, which is what his waist has become. (But don't tell him that. No reason to rile the beast.)

Another reason it's easier for men to lose weight is because they typically have more muscle than women. Muscle burns more calories than fat, so men tend to have a faster metabolism—5 to 10 percent faster than women. Plus, men have more testosterone. If they start lifting weights, they build muscle tissue much faster. (Yeah I know, biology again—annoying, but important to know.)

When it comes to food, men's and women's brains are wired differently. One study found that when people who aren't hungry are asked to smell, taste, and look at treats like chocolate, cake, and pizza, the part of the brain that controls the drive to eat lights up in women . . . but not men. Additional research has found that after exercise, ghrelin (a hormone that signals hunger) increases in women . . . but not men. Researchers theorize this is the female body's natural way to fight energy deficits that could have a negative impact on fertility. (Yes, it's unfair, ladies—biology again.)

Men also have an easier time because they typically take a more balanced approach when it comes to weight loss. They're less likely to adopt extreme measures and "quick fixes" like juices cleanses, meal skipping, or fad diets. Remember the Cabbage Soup Diet? Yuck!

Men also don't obsess about weight loss, which is a good thing.

Focusing on the scale isn't healthy, especially psychologically, and can slow weight loss progress. Weight fluctuates daily. Scales don't measure your individual percentage of muscle, bone, and body fat, or the amount of food or water you've consumed during the day. The scale won't measure positive health changes like feeling more energetic and having a lower heart rate, cholesterol level, and blood pressure.

For all these reasons, don't encourage him to weigh himself daily. Once a week is fine. If he focuses too much on the numbers between his feet and they don't go down as fast as he would like or think they should (don't we all think we should lose weight faster?), he may judge himself negatively, feel discouraged, and be tempted to give up. Don't let him—that's *exactly* what diabetes wants him to do.

Just stick to our plan. Focus on healthy eating and creative cheating and the weight loss will follow. (More on creative cheating in Chapter 12, "Mike and Ellen's Diabetes-Defeating Meal Plan.")

"I'M NOT FAT . . . I'M BIG"

Generally, men don't see themselves as fat or heavy. When women look in the mirror we see all our imperfections. We see "fat," even when we're not. When men look into the mirror they see "big," not fat. To men, big equals strong and strong equals good. Even when men recognize they're overweight, it bothers them much less than it does women. Most men don't have the negative body image issues that plague women. Fewer men feel bad about how they look, and appearance has less significant impact on male self-image, self-esteem, and confidence. There are a slew of societal, economic, and anthropological reasons for this, but that's a whole other book. Right now, we just want to get him healthy. You can enlighten him after defeating diabetes.

Men tend to focus on exercise rather than substantially chang-ing their diet to lose weight, thinking they can "exercise" or "weight lift" diabetes away. Problem is, diet plays the bigger role in terms of weight loss, but guys don't realize or want to admit that. Lifting weights is macho. Eating tofu isn't. So you're going to have to educate him a bit to defeat diabetes.

A Michael Message to Your Man

Tell him not to worry, ladies. He can defeat diabetes without becoming tofu dependent if he follows our plan. When we men were younger, we could drop weight quickly just by working out. But guys, we ain't that young anymore. Our metabolism is slowing down. Now it takes more than just adding a few reps in the gym to control our weight. That's part of the reason you and I and millions of other men became susceptible to diabetes. The "I'll just work harder in the gym" mentality doesn't cut it anymore. Your *diet* needs the new workout program, not your biceps.

Another challenge is when guys *have to* lose weight they tend to go about it privately. They're less likely to use a support system (Weight Watchers, for example), which can lead them to abandon healthy eating when they feel stressed, depressed, discouraged, tired, or bored with bland diet food. Which is why we don't advocate "diet food" when it comes to defeating diabetes, as you'll see in "Mike and Ellen's Diabetes-Defeating Meal Plan" in chapter 12. Since he probably won't join a group that provides accountability and encouragement, *you* have to be his weight loss support system.

He doesn't have to eat and exercise like you to be healthy. (He won't anyway, so save your energy and ammunition for battles that matter.) Successfully helping him defeat diabetes comes from understanding his habits and motivations. Then you can work with him to follow the health strategies and tasty nutrition tactics we outline in this book and make them part of his (and your) everyday life.

Remember ladies: we are NOT talking about putting him on a diet or eating diet foods. In fact, don't even use the word "diet" around him. *Real men don't diet. Real men get in shape.* So let him have his little fantasy and we'll just call this his Factory-Recommended

50,000 Mile Tune-Up and Engine Flush. That sounds macho enough, doesn't it?

10 SIMPLE WEIGHT LOSS STRATEGIES YOU CAN START RIGHT NOW

Here are 10 simple things you can do right now to help him lose weight and get a jump on defeating this disease.

1. Have Him Eat a Healthy Breakfast

Eating a healthy, nutrient-packed breakfast that includes protein, whole grains, and fruit will help keep his blood sugar levels steady all morning and control hunger, preventing him from overeating later in the day. New research shows that eating more calories at breakfast and less at dinner can help suppress glucose surges throughout the day.

2. Slow Down

Encourage him to eat slowly and savor his food. Limit eating on the run as much as possible. It takes the brain about 20 minutes after the stomach is full to realize it is, in fact, full. Eating fast usually means eating too much.

3. Healthy Snacking

Pack him healthy snacks (such as yogurt and fruit or an ounce of almonds) to take to work. Makes it a lot easier to ignore the donut platter in the break room. We provide plenty of healthy snack options in chapter 8.

4. Make Friends with H_2O

One of the easiest ways to help him reduce the number of calories he's consuming is to cut out high-calorie beverages like soda and sports drinks. No diet soda either. Studies show diet drinks may increase his cravings for sweets and high-calorie foods. (The brain anticipates and expects the calories detected by the sweet taste and adjusts appetite accordingly.) Replace these caloric catastrophes with good old free, zero-calorie water.

5. Start Small

Slow and steady wins the weight loss race and is key to reducing his set point so he can lose weight AND keep it off—forever! So start small. Shoot for reducing his daily intake by 300 calories, as we discussed in chapter 1. Once he sees how easy that is, he will be more receptive to continuing with the plan.

The Many Benefits of H_2O

Have your partner drink a glass of water prior to his meal. It will fill him up so he will eat less during the meal. Many people mix up hunger and thirst signals, so drinking water can curtail calorie intake. The body is about 60 percent water, so drinking water maintains the proper balance of body fluids, which is key for digestion, circulation, nutrient transportation, and maintaining body temperature. Plus, drinking water will energize his muscles, help his kidneys and digestive track work properly, and keep his skin looking good.

---

6. Healthy Up Happy Hour

It's fine to enjoy a drink or two, but be aware that calories in drinks vary widely. That piña colada has nearly 500 calories, while a 12-ounce can of light beer has only about 100. To keep his calories under control, encourage him to stick to light beer, wine (about 125 calories per glass), or spirits (1.5 ounces of vodka, rum, tequila, or whiskey only have about 100 calories) without caloric mixers such as sodas or fruit juices.

7. Pile on the Veggies

Veggies fill you up without filling you out, plus they displace high-caloric items on the plate! Save 100 to 200 calories by replacing some of his starchy pasta, rice, or potatoes with a cup of veggies. Do it every day and after six months you've saved approximately 27,000 calories. That's about 15 pounds a year! Even if you just replace half the starch with veggies it's a great first step. Like we've been saying, calories add up. Slow, steady, and consistent calorie reduction—not elimination, just *reduction*—wins this race and reverses diabetes.

8. Remove Temptation to Snack at Night

"I generally avoid temptation unless I can't resist it." —Mae West

Evening is the worst time for him to eat. Calories eaten at night have a more negative impact on blood sugar than calories eaten earlier in the day. So close down the kitchen after dinner. Have small indulgences such as a favorite fruit or a few cups of air-popped popcorn available for evening snacking. (Save time, money, and calories over expensive, fat-laden, store-bought popcorn by popping your own at home.) Remember, we men are simple creatures. What's not there we can't eat. What is there we will eat.

9. Shop Slim

Instead of eliminating his favorite foods, which will only cause strife and lead to behind-the-back cheat eating, buy smaller amounts and limit portions. For example, leave one or two cookies on a plate instead of the whole box on the counter. Or buy small, single-serving bags of chips instead of bags big enough to feed an entire Boy Scout troop. (This is called "surreptitious portion control." More on this technique in chapter 8.)

10. Get Creative

Cutting down on calories isn't just about weighing and measuring; it's also about being creative. For example, buy smaller plates. It's a weird trick, but studies show people eat less when the plate is smaller because it seems like there's more food on the plate. Or serve spicy food—it will boost his metabolism and decrease his appetite.

Remember, health benefits appear when he's lost just 5 to 10 percent of his body weight. All it takes are a few simple changes. Nothing dramatic, no food denial, no starvation diets . . . and he didn't have to eat one piece of tofu! See, it's really not that hard.

Chapter 4

Discovering His Food Personality

Your husband's "food personality" and eating habits played a significant role in developing diabetes. Now, we're going to show you how to manage and redirect his food personality to help defeat diabetes.

Most men fall into one or more of the following five food personality categories. Where does your hubby fit?

1. THE SNEAKY SNACKER: A FLEET FOOD FELON

He snacks throughout the day, usually on unhealthy, high-calorie foods. Snacking is a complex behavior that's motivated by a number of factors. It can be triggered by seeing food (either real or an advertisement), boredom, being too hungry, not eating the right foods, and uncomfortable emotions.

Whereas snacking in moderation on healthy foods like fruits and vegetables, low-fat dairy products, nuts, and whole grains can help people with diabetes stay fueled and keep their blood sugar levels steady, unconscious unhealthy snacking (chips late at night or a fistful of candy at 3:00 p.m.) can lead to increased blood sugar levels and weight gain.

The key is to help your sneaky snacker understand why he's snacking. One of the most powerful ways to do this is to teach him to pause before he eats *anything* and ask himself one simple question: Am I hungry? This crucial step will help him recognize the difference between actual, real hunger and mere cravings, which are a manifestation of desire, not actual hunger.

Here are some of the most common sneaky snacker scenarios, along with tactics to counteract his unhealthy munching.

He Skips Meals

Does he skip meals and power through work on coffee, not eating enough during the day? Is he using candy and sugary carbs to keep his energy up? No wonder he's ravenous by the end of work, ready to gobble anything he can get his hands on the minute he comes home.

The solution here is to get him to eat regular, small meals and keep healthy, energizing snacks on hand during the day when his body needs the fuel. Bagging his lunch and snacks from home not only saves money but ensures he will maintain balanced, healthy blood sugar levels throughout the day.

He's Bored

Sneaky snackers often eat when they are bored because eating is a pleasant way to pass time. The key here is to help him recognize that he's not snacking because he's hungry—he's snacking for entertainment. Short-term fun . . . yes. Long-term health problems leading to nerve damage, stroke, and heart disease . . . also yes. Seems like a pretty steep price to pay for a snack. Together, develop activities other than eating that will relieve his boredom, such as taking a walk, reading a book, practicing a hobby, learning a new skill, or seeking new challenges.

It's His Routine

Is snacking part of his routine? Does he grab a donut every time he passes the break room at work? Buy chips and soda at the mini-mart when he fills up the car? Can't watch a movie without a tub of buttered death in his lap? (The popcorn isn't the problem. It's all the fat they laden it with.)

It's time to break this routine. Gently, remind him to stay out of the break room. Fill up the car yourself so he has no reason to stop. Bring a small bag of healthy nuts, air-popped popcorn, or baked corn chips for him to munch at the movies.

He's Feeling Down

Negative emotions such as feeling lonely, sad, or angry often lead to snacking. If he's snacking to blunt the impact of uncomfortable emotions, he's a combo snacker-emotional eater. Check out our advice for the final food personality type, the emotional eater, below.

He Succumbs to Late-Night Snack Attacks

Research shows that nocturnal munching is triggered by the body's internal clock, called the circadian system, which increases hunger and cravings for sweet, starchy, and salty foods in the evenings. While the urge to consume more in the evenings helped our ancestors store energy to survive during times of famine, in our modern, high-calorie environment, late-night snacking results in weight gain, higher blood sugar levels, and diabetes. To make matters worse, the body becomes more insulin-resistant (less able to use blood sugar) at night. Kicking his late-night snack addiction will go a long way toward helping him defeat diabetes.

If you've got a midnight muncher on your hands, you need to shift his focus away from late-night food. Here are some tips:

✓ *Skip the food porn and turn off the tube.* TV food ads are designed to make people feel hungry. Don't let him watch them. Watch a video, DVR your programs, or suggest he get up and stretch or walk around the house during commercials. Michael gets up and does quick, two-minute chores like taking the garbage out, doing a few dishes, or playing with the dog.

✓ *Help him wind down.* If he's eating because he's bored, restless, or has trouble sleeping, help him recognize what he's going through and then help him make a conscious choice to do something other than eating to relax. (We provide specific ways to bust stress and relax in chapter 5.)

✓ *Change his routine.* The classic example is to have him brush his teeth right after dinner. You'd be surprised how effective this little psychological trick is. People are much less likely to eat after brushing.

✓ *Get him to bed.* Try and get him to come to bed with you so he doesn't stay up and snack while you sleep.

"That was my old trick—tuck Ellen in, then tuck into some fun food and late-night TV. Not anymore!"

✓ *Remove the temptation.* One of the most effective ways to control a sneaky snacker is also one of the simplest: keep tempting snack foods out of the house. (You'll see this repeated often because it's so important . . . and easy to do.)

2. THE VOLUME EATER: HE LIKES TO TURN IT UP TO 11

Volume or big eaters consume very large amounts of food that's usually high in calories. Doesn't matter what it is as long as there's lots of it . . . and there are seconds. As a result, their weight remains stubbornly fixed at a high point, which keeps their blood sugar levels elevated. In addition, when large volumes of food are dumped into his digestive system, it propels his already unhealthy blood sugar levels even higher, making diabetes worse.

Volume eaters often eat rapidly, spending less than 20 minutes on meals. This conveyor belt fashion of ingesting leaves them way over their suggested calorie and carb allotment for the day . . . sometimes in just one meal.

Don't berate him or make him feel bad for overeating. Offer loving support. Understanding is key. Many volume eaters have larger than average stomachs and lower levels of appetite-suppressing hormones, making it easier for them to consume lots of food. Being diagnosed with diabetes is often the turning point volume eaters need to finally decide to save themselves and stop their destructive behavior. Getting the big eater to go easy isn't easy, but the stakes are great.

"I'll have mine medium rare . . . Just joking, ladies."

Here's how to help your volume eater:

Set a Speed Trap

No more accelerating past the FULL sign. He needs to pump the brakes on his eating speed. Remind him to *pause* throughout meals to give his brain time to catch up and signal that his stomach is full. Encourage him to chew every bite and *enjoy* his food. Suggest he put down his fork and take a sip of water between bites. Reassure him there's no need to hurry. Make meals pleasant with light conversation. (Meals are not the time to talk about Junior's bad grades.) Changing his eating speed will take time, so be patient and offer gentle reminders and encouragement.

Discourage Seconds

Better yet, make less so there aren't seconds, or immediately put the food away after you cook it so it can be eaten at another meal.

If he *thinks* he's hungry after his serving, help him get into the habit of doing something—chores, a work project, a hobby—for 20 minutes right after dinner (i.e., distract him). This method will give his body time to send signals of satiety to his brain before overconsumption occurs.

Downsize the Dish

To defeat diabetes and save his life, dish out his food for him (at least initially), until he learns how much he can and should eat. And use smaller dishes. Numerous studies have shown that larger-sized portions, food packages, plates, and tableware lead to higher consumption of food and drink. One study found that simply shifting from a 12-inch to a 10-inch plate resulted in a 22 percent decrease in calories consumed. He'll feel more satisfied because his mind will think he's eating a full plate.

Believe it or not, the color of dishes matters too. Make sure the color of the dishes is different than the color of the food you serve (e.g., don't serve pasta with red sauce on a red plate or pasta with Alfredo sauce on a white plate). When there is no contrast between plate color and food color, serving sizes look small so he'll feel deprived and want to eat more.

Pump It Up!

"Only have a little" does not compute for volume eaters, so you've got to decrease the number of calories on his plate without noticeably decreasing his volume of food. You do this by increasing nutrition density (adding healthy foods like veggies that are low in calories) and decreasing caloric density (reducing high-calorie foods, especially fats). The result? His hunger will be satisfied with fewer calories consumed, leading to . . . wait for it . . . weight loss! Plenty more tips on exactly how to "pump it up" in chapters 8 and 12.

Dull His Hunger

Start meals with a big salad and two glasses of water. His stomach will feel almost full before he's even had a chance to tuck into the main event.

---

3. THE NEANDERTHAL: HE'S IN A SERIOUS RELATIONSHIP WITH MEAT

Lucky for your carnivorous caveman, meat won't increase his blood sugar, but the extra calories do hinder weight loss, which makes it harder to control diabetes. Research shows eating too much meat, especially the processed kind increases your risk of cardiovascular disease and cancer.

So take a look at how much lunch meat, hot dogs, sausage, and bacon he's eating, then come up with ways to substitute healthier meats. For example, try sliced turkey instead of salami or bologna, or chicken sausages instead of full-fat pork sausages. These products are delicious, and if you don't make a big deal about it he probably won't even notice. If he still wants a bologna sandwich, cut down on the slices and try to limit the processed meats to no more than one meal a week. Try roasting a whole chicken (or buying a rotisserie chicken if you're short on time) or turkey (it's not just for Thanksgiving!) and slicing it for tasty, healthful sandwiches during the week. By cutting back on the fatty meats during the week, he can still enjoy an occasional Brontosaurus Burger over the weekend.

4. THE JUNK FOOD JUNKIE WANTS HIS FAST FOOD FIX

"Here, I made you a three-bean salad for lunch."

"Don't bother, honey. I'll just grab some fried dough at Captain Cupcake's Cholesterol Café drive-thru window."

If you're man is addicted to junk food, he's not alone. North Americans spend about *$124 billion* a year on snack foods. Cheese puffs, potato chips, fried foods, and drive-thru cheeseburgers are designed to taste great and induce the desire to eat more—way more. These foods are eaten quickly and literally melt in your mouth, tricking your brain into thinking you haven't consumed much while you stuff yourself with more and more sugar, salt, fat, and calories.

Junk food is a big problem for people with diabetes or prediabetes. Because it's loaded with simple carbohydrates and generally low in fiber and protein, junk food creates huge spikes in blood sugar levels. The high calorie count leads to weight gain as unhealthy food additives and salt stimulate taste buds so he wants more . . . and more.

If he's a junk food junkie, simply cutting out the crap may be enough to help him lose a significant amount of weight and get his blood sugar under control. Yes, defeating diabetes can be this simple! Here are some ways to get started . . .

Pump Up His Motivation

No junkie kicks a habit without clear, personal motivation and self-interest. Explain to him that junking the junk food will have a significant, immediate, positive effect on his diabetes, heart, and cardiovascular system. The resulting weight loss will have him feeling and looking better than he has in years. Plus, he'll be setting a good health and fitness example for everyone around him.

Hopefully, he will come to understand (or you might have to beat it into his head) that improving his health, happiness, confidence and self-esteem is more important than another bag of diabetes-inducing sludge roiling his blood sugar, clogging his arteries, and eventually killing him. That's not hyperbole—the junk food really will take years off his life if he can't kick junk off the menu NOW!

Inventory His Junk

Have him save the wrappers and receipts his habit generates. Doing so will help him see clearly just how much junk he's eating and how much he's paying to ruin his own health.

Cut Back Slowly

While some men can go cold turkey, cutting all the junk at once can be tough for others to handle. If he needs to go slow, then each week have him cut the amount of junk he's eating in half. After a few weeks he'll be almost done with junk food forever.

Remove Temptation

Yes, we say this often, but it works. Outta sight is outta mind. So get the junk out of the house and remind him to keep the chips and candy out of his desk drawer at work.

Provide Alternatives

If he likes salty, crunchy foods, send him to work with individually portioned bags of light popcorn, baby carrots with a little hummus for dipping, or some nuts. If he has a sweet tooth, pack him his favorite fruit or bake a batch of our high-protein, high-fiber, diabetic-friendly cookies.

Order Right

As we've discussed, avoid highly processed foods that contain large amounts of refined sugar, salt, and additives. Many fast food restaurants have healthy options such as chicken wraps and salads that easily fit into a diabetic-friendly meal plan. To ensure that he orders healthy options, look at fast food menus together online before he hits the drive-thru. No healthy options? Don't eat there. (More on ordering healthy fast food in chapter 9.)

Avoid the Hungries!

Don't let hunger trigger a relapse for your recovering junkie! Letting your man get too hungry can trigger a junk food binge, so plan meals and snacks to avoid this outcome. Make sure he has a healthy breakfast that's packed with protein and fiber so he doesn't get hungry later. Encourage him to eat small, healthy snacks at least every three hours to keep his hunger (and blood sugar) under control.

Treat Him with a Treat

Remember, weaning him off junk food is a process, so allow for an occasional decadent treat once or twice a week (even if it is a slice of pepperoni pizza). All foods can be eaten on our plan. In fact, having small amounts of the foods he loves can really help him stick with his diet during the rest of the week. As he cuts out the junk, he'll find that he enjoys and appreciates the occasional treat even more.

5. THE EMOTIONAL EATER: HE USES FOOD TO COMBAT STRESS

"Emotions? I'll have mine with onion rings." —A Guy

Many people are emotional eaters, using food to mitigate or hide from stressful issues or turmoil. Like our junk food junkie above, most emotional eaters don't realize they are overeating for the wrong reasons. They mindlessly eat to soothe and distract themselves when they're upset or stressed. And of course the more upset they get, the harder it is for them to avoid emotional eating. Food is their mood-enhancing drug of choice.

Emotional eating does offer a source of distraction from what's bothering him . . . for a while. But when the food's gone he's still left with the uncomfortable emotions, because food doesn't resolve anything. It just diverts his attention for the moment. Fortunately, there are a number of things you can do to help your emotional eater.

Write It Down

The first step is building self-awareness. Keep a food journal for three days (two workdays and one weekend day). Ask him to write down what, where, when, and why he eats, how hungry he is before eating, and how he feels during eating. This will help him recognize when he's eating to soothe emotions or distract himself and when he's eating because he's hungry. He'll start to understand what situations, specific times of day, and feelings tend to trigger his emotional eating.

Help Him Express His Feelings

Ask him to articulate what's stressing or upsetting him. If he can't change the situation (for example, a long commute to work or a boss he hates), see if he can change how he thinks about and reacts to the situation. Can he frame the commute as a time to relax by listening to music or a book on tape? Can he take steps to minimize contact with his boss during the workday?

If he reaches for the cookie jar when he's stressed, depressed, or lonely, help him become aware of his feelings and his behavior *before* the cookie gets crunched. Sometimes just taking a moment to stop and think is all he will need to walk away. The more aware he becomes of his inner experience, the more he can find healthier ways to cope with his feelings. The solution to emotional eating is not food control; it's emotional control and self-knowledge. Control emotion and you control calories. Control calories and you control diabetes. Yes, it really is that simple! (We say this a lot because it's true.)

Teach Him to Eat Mindfully

Once he becomes aware of his emotional eating patterns, the next step is to help him eat with awareness. Encourage him to remove distractions (such as the computer screen or television) while eating. At home, teach him to chew his food slowly, use all five senses to thoroughly enjoy his meals, and eat just until he's satisfied, not stuffed. Over time he'll learn the difference between physical hunger and emotional hunger and how not to overfill his tank.

Make Him HALT

Finally, teach your emotional eater the acronym HALT, which stands for hungry, angry, lonely, and tired. Help him recognize the feeling of true hunger, which should be the only signal to give his body fuel that he listens to. Sit down and create a list of things that he can do (other than eating!) and ways you can help him when he's feeling angry, lonely, or tired. Discover what is causing his anger and explore ways he can avoid, properly express, or transform it. If loneliness is an issue, encourage him to reach out and connect with others who want to see him happy and healthy. If he's tired, make sure he gets good sleep.

Your husband's food personality type doesn't have to define him and his eating habits. Follow our suggestions and he will be so surprised by how well you understand and love him that he may change his food personality without any resistance at all.

Chapter 5

Rewiring His Brain for Weight Loss
Using Psychology to Defeat Diabetes

Adopting a diabetes-free lifestyle isn't simply a matter of changing what's in the refrigerator and cupboards. Real change requires sustained effort and staying positive. This is where behavior modification can have its greatest, life-changing impact. Behavior modification techniques will help you and him maintain the life-saving, diabetes-defeating lifestyle changes the two of you are working on and help him maintain a positive outlook as the pounds flee and his health returns!

Best of all, you don't need to be a psychologist to effectively use these techniques. We're going to show you how.

CHANGE AGENT . . . YOU

Begging won't work. Nagging won't work. Hollering, screaming, or forcing in any way won't work. So what works? It's actually quite simple: encouragement. Yes, encouragement, support, and what we shrinks call "behavior modification."

Behavior modification is a series of psychological techniques you can use to get your husband to do what you want him to do. (Yes, you can modify some of these techniques to get him to leave the toilet seat down.) In contrast to diets and drugs, which offer quick but temporary (sometimes toxic) solutions, behavior change leads to permanent transformation because it helps him to gradually establish new, healthier habits and make them part of his daily life . . . subconsciously.

The crux of behavior modification is this: To get your man to modify bad habits and add new, healthy ones, *reward desirable behaviors* and *discourage undesirable behaviors* on a regular basis. For example, when he eats a healthy breakfast, works out, or snacks on fruit instead of candy, give him a kiss and a kind, encouraging word. Look him in the eye and tell him what an amazing person he is. Make him feel good and express how happy he's making *you* by getting healthy. In other words, get him to associate healthy habits with *praise*.

Reward him consistently, every time he does a positive behavior.

"Ellen, it sounds like you're training a dog."
"If the collar fits, Fido . . ."

When he slips back into unhealthy behaviors such as eating chips while watching television, turn off the TV for a moment and ask him why he isn't keeping his promise to only eat at the kitchen table. See how you've discouraged the negative behavior without actually criticizing him (or hitting him on the nose with a rolled-up newspaper)? All you're doing is asking, nicely, for an explanation. Often this simple nudge is enough for him to drop the chips and get back on track. If he balks, remind him that you love him and want him around for a long, long time.

Here are five behavior modification techniques you can use right now to help him systematically modify his eating, exercise, and other behaviors.

---

1. BREAKING BAD: PUT THE BRAKES ON NEGATIVE BEHAVIOR BY BUILDING AWARENESS WITH SELF-MONITORING

First, we gotta break the bad before we can build the good. Every bad habit—from nail biting and leaving the toilet seat up to smoking and overeating—can be broken. The key is to first make the person with the bad habit *aware* of the bad habit. That's where self-monitoring comes in.

Self-monitoring is a powerful, positive, bad habit–breaking behavior modification tool that builds self-awareness, self-esteem, and self-confidence. Essentially, self-monitoring is observing, measuring, recording, and evaluating one's own actions. When practiced intentionally and consistently, self-monitoring will enable your partner to learn from his mistakes, change his behavior, and avoid future slipups. Research shows that when used on a regular basis, self-monitoring, especially keeping consistent food records, significantly boosts weight loss success.

With self-monitoring, he will start to understand his behaviors (i.e., what, when, and how much he eats) as well as what supports and, more importantly, what gets in the way of positive change. Building greater awareness will help him find better ways to maintain new behaviors when his initial, fear-based motivation (triggered by his diagnosis of diabetes or pre diabetes) starts to fade. This will help prevent depression and defeatism when he hits a plateau and temporarily stops losing weight, which happens to *everyone*. Plus, self-monitoring provides valuable records that will give you both a concrete way to measure the arc of his success in defeating diabetes.

Here are four key categories that he can easily monitor to improve his health and defeat diabetes:

Food

Keeping food records is a powerful behavior modification technique. To start, have him set a goal to keep food records (more on goal setting in a moment) and reward him when he does so. Have him write down what, when, and how much he eats and how hungry he is before and after meals and snacks.

He can write it on a spreadsheet, his cell phone, or good ol' pen and paper. Whatever he finds comfortable. At the end of the day, encourage him to review what he ate (recorded) and think about what went well and how he could do better tomorrow. If he had a perfect healthy eating day, congratulate him, encourage him to feel good about himself, and find an appropriate reward for his accomplishment.

Physical Activity

There are numerous ways to measure physical activity. If you want to go all out, you can buy him a fitness or activity tracker that he can wear around his wrist. Depending on the model, it can measure everything from heart rate and calories burned to inactivity time and quality of sleep. A less expensive option is a pedometer, which measures and records how many steps he takes and the total mileage he covers. If he can work up to 5,000 steps (about 2½ miles) per day, that's great! Sure it sounds like a lot, but when you break it up into smaller walks throughout the day, you'd be surprised how manageable it is. For example, parking his car at the end of the company lot instead of at the door can add a quarter mile per day in steps. How about using the stairs instead of the elevator at work? That's more steps, more mileage, more positive results.

Weight

We don't recommend daily weigh-ins because it can create an unhealthy obsession with weight. We do, however, encourage weekly weigh-ins to help him monitor his progress. Once a week, have him record changes in his weight from the previous week, and graph the changes as a reminder of how well he's doing with his weight loss program.

If he doesn't want to share his weight with you, that's okay. He might be embarrassed by the number, or discouraged if he thinks he's not losing weight fast enough, or feel his weight is private information.

Michael doesn't like to weigh himself. His alternative to the scale? He tracked his progress via belt notches and changes in clothing size. The important thing is that your mate (or you if he won't) keeps a record and reviews it. This subtle form of behavior modification is a powerful tool to keep him on track.

Sleep (This Is One for You to Monitor)

Diabetes can cause sleep problems. Conversely, sleep problems can make diabetes worse and lead to weight gain. When blood sugar levels are high, people don't sleep as well, and they urinate more because the kidneys are trying to expel the excess sugar, which interrupts sleep. Plus, fatigue can trigger overeating as people try to increase their energy by consuming food. Please, monitor your man and make sure he gets seven to eight hours of quality sleep every night.

Here are a few sleep tips:

✓ *Ditch the drinks.* Remind him to stop drinking caffeine in the afternoon and alcohol late in the evening. Both interfere with sleep.

✓ *Lighten the meals.* Indigestion can make it hard to sleep, so avoid heavy meals at night.

✓ *Cool the room.* Keep your bedroom cool (60° to 67° is best). Body temperature drops as you fall asleep, so cooling down the room jump-starts the process.

✓ *Dim the lights.* Make sure the room is dark. Light inhibits the secretion of melatonin, a hormone that promotes sleep.

---

2. GOAL SETTING: CHARTING HIS ROAD MAP TO SUCCESS

Goal setting is crucial to accomplishing great things in life . . . including defeating diabetes. Goals are powerful behavior change tools because they give you something to plan and work for, which propels you forward. They transform what feels like insurmountable mountains (losing 30 pounds) into a series of manageable hills (losing 1 to 2 pounds per week). Goals help you believe in yourself, stay accountable, and live life to the fullest. Plus, setting goals is key to creating healthy habits.

To help hubby understand the importance of goals, use a sports analogy: without goals, you spend your life running up and down the field and never score! Help him set both specific, short-term weekly goals and long-term (three month, six month, one year) goals.

To be successful, goals MUST be written down. This is a form of commitment that will keep him on track. Remember these four points when setting goals . . .

Goals MUST Be Specific

For example, "I'll walk more" isn't good enough. "I'll walk four days per week during my lunch break" is specific. The more specific a goal, the more likely he is to achieve it.

Goals Must Be Realistic

While ambitious goals are good, being too ambitious can be discouraging. One of the best ways to improve his belief that he can defeat diabetes is to have some early successes. Start with small, concrete, achievable goals that are easy to attain. This will help build his confidence so he can tackle more ambitious goals in the future.

Goals Require Feedback and Reinforcement

Discussing how he's doing will improve his progress. Keep the feedback positive. If you have negative feedback, make it constructive with positive suggestions to help him get back on track. Instead of saying, "I can't believe you ate the whole cheesecake," try, "Why did you feel the need to eat all the cheesecake?" See the difference? The first response ends the conversation. The latter response *starts* a conversation.

Broaden his circle of support beyond you. Encourage him to seek feedback from his doctor, other family members, or anyone he trusts and respects. Friends can provide excellent motivation . . . but beware—some may try to undermine his success because they have weight or health issues of their own they aren't addressing, or they fear his getting healthy will change their relationship.

"Mike, how come you don't come to the all-you-can-eat buffet at Freddie's Fry Shack for lunch anymore? You mad at us?"

"No biggie, Bob. I just don't want to die anytime soon."

Goals Must Be SMART

SMART stands for Specific, Measurable, Achievable, Relevant, and Time-bound. To help your husband set SMART goals, sit down together and ask him these five questions:

- To be **S**pecific ask: What exactly do you want to accomplish?

- To be **M**easurable ask: How will you determine whether or not you've reached your goal?

- To be **A**chievable ask: How sure are you on a scale of 1 (won't be able to achieve it) to 10 (100 percent sure) that you can do this? The best goals are around an 8—challenging, yet doable.

- To be **Relevant** ask: How important is this goal to you, your health and defeating diabetes?

- To be **Time-bound** ask: When will you know you have accomplished your goal?

Examples of SMART short-term goals are:

- ❑ I will walk for 30 minutes, five days per week.
- ❑ I will keep food records five days per week by writing down everything I eat on Monday, Wednesday, Thursday, Friday, and Sunday.
- ❑ I will bring a bag lunch to work four days per week instead of ordering takeout.
- ❑ I will eat a healthy breakfast five days a week that consists of two servings of whole grains (e.g., 100 percent whole-wheat bread), a piece of fruit, and a cup of low-fat milk or yogurt.
- ❑ At work I will eat a cheese stick and a piece of fruit for my late-afternoon snack instead of a candy bar.
- ❑ I will limit the number of carbs I eat at dinner every night to no more than 60 grams. (We'll show you exactly how to determine amounts like this in chapter 6.)
- ❑ Four days per week I will have an apple for my evening snack.

Examples of SMART long-term goals are:

- ❑ I will lose 10 pounds in three months.
- ❑ I will get my LDL (i.e., "bad") cholesterol down to under 100.
- ❑ I will reduce my A1C (a test for diabetics that gives a picture of the average amount of glucose in the blood over the last three months) by at least 25 percent before my next doctor's visit in six months.
- ❑ In three months I will be able to walk one mile in under 20 minutes.

Setting long-term goals is important. They increase focus and motivation by giving him a clear path to follow . . . the road map to success he needs to defeat diabetes.

3. STIMULUS CONTROL: AN OUNCE OF PREVENTION IS WORTH A POUND OF CURE!

Stimulus control is a term that describes situations in which a specific behavior is triggered by the presence of some stimulus. For example, if hubby sees a Domino's commercial and orders a large sausage and pepperoni with extra cheese, the commercial is a stimulus for eating pizza. Remove the stimulus (e.g., turn the TV off or watch a DVD) and you change his behavior.

To better understand stimulus control and how to use it to change his eating habits, it's helpful to consider the ABCs of behavior: antecedents, behavior, and consequences. Antecedents are simply the events, feelings, and situations that occur *before* the behavior. The behavior refers to the eating episode and the related events and feelings that occur around or *during* the behavior. The consequences are the events, feelings, and attitudes that occur *after* the behavior.

The ABCs of eating behavior typically occur in steps . . .

First comes the antecedents or stimulus: You buy a large, 24-ounce bag of chips plus dip because you expect guests this weekend. You leave the bag on the counter, forgetting to put it away because you're in a rush to pick up the kids. He's bored and home alone. He turns on the TV. There's a game on. (As Michael told you earlier, there's *always* a game on ESPN.) He goes into the kitchen. His hungry eyes settle on the beautiful yellow and blue bag of his favorite fun food. He's only going to have "a couple." Yeah, right . . . that's why he takes the whole bag into the TV room—so he can only have "a couple."

Next comes the behavior: he eats half the bag while watching TV. That's an approximately 1,900 nuclear calorie bomb with 180 blood sugar–busting grams of carbs.

And finally the consequences: he feels like a stuffed, guilty failure . . . further weakening his resolve. "What an idiot. I ate half the bag. Well, damage done, might as well finish them . . ."

To change his behavior and help him form new habits, you must break the links in the ABC chain. In other words, remove the triggers or antecedents. For example, to stop the behavior, don't buy potato chips, or put them away where he won't see them. Remind him of his promises to only eat in the kitchen and write down what he eats.

Avoiding the stimulus (TV and potato chips) is the most important tactic, because it prevents the negative behavior from happening so new, positive behaviors can flourish.

4. COGNITIVE RESTRUCTURING: MOLDING HIS MIND TO DEFEAT DIABETES

The body achieves what the mind believes. We create our life with our thoughts, feelings, and beliefs, which is why his mind is a powerful weapon in the fight against diabetes. If he thinks he will be successful at losing weight, controlling his blood sugar, and defeating diabetes, he will change his behavior to coincide with his beliefs. Conversely, if he thinks he's doomed to a life of toxic drugs, amputations, and diabetic disability, that is what he will create.

Fortunately, with a little work and help from you, he can develop a positive, diabetes-defeating mindset . . . and keep his toes.

Cognitive restructuring can help him learn to identify, dispute, and restructure his counterproductive, negative thoughts and replace them with positive, diabetes-defeating, useful thoughts.

Think of cognitive restructuring as a renovation project for the mind. You're not getting a new one; you're just fixing up the perfectly good one you already have so it works better. You build a new mind by tearing down old, negative thoughts and beliefs and replacing them with new, positive ones. The new, positive thoughts will build positive emotions and lead to the positive health behaviors that will reverse diabetes. Plus, just like renovating a room makes you happier and more comfortable, his renovated mindset will make him an overall happier and healthier person—a great bonus for you!

Here are two powerful cognitive restructuring techniques he can use right now to defeat diabetes.

Notice His Negative Thoughts

The first step in cognitive restructuring is to teach him to notice his negative thoughts. Unhelpful thoughts like "I'm too fat to get in shape," "Nothing I can do, it's a disease," or "I don't have time to exercise" will undermine his success.

When he indulges in self-defeating, negative thoughts, tell him to *stop* thinking and talking that way. Then challenge him by asking how else he could think about this, or if he can imagine a more positive outcome. For example, instead of "I'm too fat to get in shape," he could think, "Lots of people lose weight and get in shape—I can too."

Test His Negative Thoughts

With this technique, you ask him to investigate his negative thoughts and beliefs to determine if they are really true. For example, if he believes, "I don't have time to exercise," encourage him to take a 15-minute walk with you once a day for a week. BINGO—thought defeated! If he thinks, "I can't eat right," serve him a healthy meal to help him see that, yes, he *can* eat right. In other words, prove the negative thought is not reality, it's just a . . . negative thought.

To take thought testing a step further, have him evaluate his negative thoughts—for example, "I can't eat right"—by writing one column of evidence that supports the thought and one column that shows this thought isn't true. If he can't come up with evidence on his own that counter the thought, help him out. He'll quickly see the lack of real evidence to support the negative thought and plenty to support the positive thought. In other words, he *can* make healthy eating choices. (If your husband's a lawyer, don't use this technique. He'll just keep objecting that the evidence is inadmissible.)

---

5. STRESS REDUCTION: CHILLAXING FOR WEIGHT LOSS

Stress is a primary predictor of relapse, driving him back to the bad, old habits that initially triggered diabetes. Think about it: When you're stressed out and frazzled, do you eat more? Most of us do. We reach for high-calorie, fat-filled, sugar-packed foods when we're stressed because they're tasty and give us a temporary high by boosting brain levels of dopamine and endorphins, two chemicals that make us feel good.

Stress increases appetite and weight gain, especially around the middle, and it reduces metabolism. (Remember, the body reacts to stress as if there's a famine, so it slows us down to conserve fuel.) One study found that stressed individuals burned 104 fewer calories a day than those who weren't stressed. Plus, stress increases blood sugar levels and blood pressure and weakens the immune system. In other words, everything you *don't* want to happen as you fight diabetes. To help him defeat diabetes, lose weight, and restore his health, it's critical for him to minimize and control stress.

Men do not handle stress the way women do. While both men and women produce the hormones cortisol and epinephrine when stressed, women generate more of the calming, soothing, connecting hormone oxytocin in response to stress. This helps explain why women talk about what's bothering them and seek connection when stressed.

In contrast, men generally repress their feelings when stressed. They often seek an escape activity to create a relaxing diversion. That's why when they're upset, men retreat to their caves to play *Call of Duty*, watch sports, or . . . eat. While this may work for him temporarily, over time isolation and bottling up his feelings will backfire, which is why you want to help him develop better ways to deal with stress.

Does he snap at people (including you) and get angry when stressed? Then he will benefit the most from soothing activities that calm him. If he worries and feels anxious when stressed, he'll benefit from activities that help him stay focused on the present moment. If he withdraws when stressed (very typical for guys), you want to encourage him to do things that help him reengage with life.

There are several stress-reduction techniques you can use to help him right now! To find the best ways to help your man handle stress, pick one or two of the suggestions below to try each week. Not every technique works for everyone, so keep trying until you find what works for him. To make the stress-reduction technique more effective, encourage him to set a goal around it. For example, every day when I come home from work I will listen to music for 20 minutes to help me relax before dinner.

Exercise

Exercise is one of the best and healthiest ways to reduce and manage stress. If he tends to lash out when stressed, going for a brisk walk can help him reduce stress and dissipate anger. In addition, aerobic exercise (like running, biking, or walking) generates feel-good hormones called endorphins (the chemical responsible for the "runner's high") that help lower stress.

Body-mind exercises like yoga or tai chi are also excellent for reducing stress. They enhance the ability to relax and gently bring the body to a balanced, calm state. If he's open to trying yoga get him a beginner's DVD. There are also plenty of easy yoga clips on YouTube he can test-drive. Start slow and simple, and avoid advanced and power yoga classes. They will be too intense and competitive and may actually increase his stress as he tries to keep up with the 100-pound rubber band in spandex . . . also known as the yoga instructor.

Practicing martial arts—such as karate, judo, or tae kwon do—is another great, stress-reducing activity, and it may appeal more to his macho sensibilities than yoga or tai chi. The various techniques will help him release energy, frustration, and tension. In addition, improving his physicality will boost his confidence and self-esteem.

Needless to say, there are dozens of exercising options out there for him. The key is finding activities he *enjoys doing*. If he perceives exercise as drudgery he is unlikely to maintain a regular fitness schedule.

Get Outside

More than 100 research studies have shown that outdoor recreation reduces stress. Spending time in nature cultivates a positive attitude and a renewed sense of connectedness, meaning, and purpose. Plus, studies show outdoor exercise has a more beneficial psychological impact than indoor exercise in reducing depression and anxiety.

Again, there is literally an entire world of opportunities out there for him. Anything that gets him up and moving outside is a positive step forward.

Meditate

You may have a hard time imagining your husband meditating, but before you scoff at this, hear us out. Just a few minutes a day of meditation can significantly reduce stress, especially for individuals who tend to be anxious, pessimistic, or angry. Meditation preserves the aging brain and literally changes its structure. For example, meditation changes activity and connectivity in the default mode network, a part of the brain that's responsible for ruminating and worrying about the past and future.

A study conducted at the Johns Hopkins School of Medicine found that for depression and anxiety, the beneficial effects of meditation rival those of antidepressants. Research on a meditation method called Mindfulness-Based Stress Reduction (MBSR) has shown that it can reduce stress (physical and mental) and anxiety. Regular meditation will help him observe his reaction to stress and the negative mind traps that often trigger it.

He doesn't need wind chimes, incense, and some bearded guru from Kathmandu to start meditating. Encourage him to think of meditation simply as a way to sit quietly for a while and calm his racing thoughts. You can have him read the instructions below, or purchase a simple meditation CD or podcast.

Basic Meditation

Sit quietly in a place where you won't be disturbed. Take a few deep, calming breaths and close your eyes. Relax your body. Then, for 2–3, minutes focus on your breathing . . . noting each breath going in and out. If your mind starts to wander, which is totally normal, or you have difficulty settling down, silently count your breaths from 1 to 10 and repeat.

Visualization

If he finds meditation difficult, try visualization, "the winners' secret." Here's how one winner put it:

"I had a clear vision of myself winning the Mr. Universe contest. It was a very spiritual thing, in a way, because I had such faith in the route,

the path, that there was never a question in my mind that I would make it." —Arnold Schwarzenegger

Visualization works because imagining something stimulates the same part of the brain as actually performing the action itself. If you're having troubling getting your man to experiment with visualization, tell him that top athletes use the technique all the time to improve confidence and performance. If he doesn't believe you, maybe he'll listen to "the Greatest" himself:

"To be a great champion you must believe you are the best. If you're not, pretend you are." —Muhammad Ali

Like meditation, visualization does not require mystic beliefs or exotic paraphernalia to perform. All it requires is a quiet place to sit where he won't be disturbed. See below for how to do it.

Deep Breathing

This is a super easy and quick stress-reduction technique that he can do anytime. The practice is powerful because it stimulates what's called the "parasympathetic" nervous system, which calms down the fight-or-flight response that is a natural human reaction to stress, and brings the body and mind back to a calm state.

Deep breathing is literally nothing more than that: breathing deeply. The quick instructions below show just how easy it is.

Visualization to Reduce Stress and Anxiety

Close your eyes and imagine visiting a calm, peaceful scene such as a lake, the beach, or the mountains. Engage as many of your senses as you can, including smell, sight, sound, and touch. Continue to experience the peaceful place in your mind for five minutes, or until you feel calm and relaxed.

Deep Breathing

Sit in a comfortable position. Relax your shoulders and close your eyes. Take a breath, then breathe out slowly through your nose for a count of five. At the end of the out breath, pause for two counts. Then inhale slowly to the count of five, expanding your belly as you breathe in. Repeat for 5–10 breaths.

QUICK AND FUN STRESS BUSTERS

Exercise and various ways to calm his mind are just the start. Here are a handful of other specific, quick ways to lower his stress levels and improve his outlook and health.

- ✓ *Listen to music.* Relaxing music has been shown to reduce the stress-inducing hormone cortisol.

- ✓ *Have silly fun.* Rent a silly movie, hit a comedy club, or watch funny pet videos on YouTube. Research shows that even anticipating laughter can reduce stress hormones.

- ✓ *Massage.* Give your man a rub. It's a fantastic way to relieve stress because physical touch generates the feel-good chemical oxytocin. The benefits are also cumulative, meaning the more he gets rubbed the better he'll feel. Which leads us to . . .

- ✓ *Have SEX.* (Are we being too subtle here?) Not only will it get his mind off what's stressing him, research shows sex can decrease symptoms of stress and lower blood pressure. Hugging increases the level of the calming chemical oxytocin, and kissing releases chemicals that ease stress hormones. So pucker up for hubby's health!

- ✓ *Eat right.* Stress depletes many essential nutrients. The right foods actually help reduce stress. Make sure he's eating foods that are high in B vitamins. Good sources include fish, poultry, green leafy vegetables, eggs and chickpeas. (Follow our meal plan guide in chapter 12 and he'll get all the Bs he needs.) It's also important to get enough vitamin C (found in citrus fruits and peppers), omega-3 fatty acids (fish), and magnesium (dark leafy greens again; nuts). Go easy on the caffeine; too much can increase stress and deplete the body of essential nutrients.

Don't worry if he's resistant to behavior modification at first. There's a good chance he will be. That's why we've given you plenty of different strategies and techniques to use. Helping him change his behavior takes time. Defeating diabetes isn't a sprint; it's a marathon. He doesn't have to come in first. He just has to finish the course.

Chapter 6

Scoring a Weight Loss Triple Play with Your Hubby's Health

This chapter will cover everything you need to know about carbohydrates, protein, and fat. You'll learn how to help hubby modify all three to lose weight, lower blood sugar, and control and eventually defeat diabetes. We'll use a sports analogy—a baseball triple play—to make it fun and easy for him to understand.

THE TRIPLE PLAY: THE ROLE OF CARBOHYDRATES, PROTEIN, AND FAT

Macronutrients are substances that are essential to our health and growth, and calories come from three of them: carbohydrates, proteins, and fats. Your body needs all three to be healthy.

In a nutshell, carbohydrates fuel body and brain. Protein is essential for growth, repair, and body regulation. Fat provides energy, keeps the immune system healthy, and helps you absorb nutrients. It also maintains cell membranes and helps regulate body temperature.

Some foods provide mostly one macronutrient. For example, chicken breast is almost all protein, rice is mostly carbs, and butter is . . . you guessed it, almost all fat. Other foods such as pizza, burritos, or beef stew are a combination of all three. Achieving the right amount of calories and balance of carbs, protein, and fat is key for losing weight, lowering his blood sugar level, and defeating diabetes.

We could spend the rest of the book explaining how carbs, protein, and fats interact in your body and how to balance them for weight loss. Yep, it is confusing. And frankly, boring.

"I don't find it boring, Michael."

"You're a dietitian, honey. You like talking about this stuff. Folks at home just want us to tell them how to lose the weight and defeat diabetes."

"You mean they aren't interested in the metabolic rate of conversion or fat absorption ratios?"

"That's exactly what I mean. So let's just tell them what they need to feed their man so he loses weight and feels great. Save the science for your next research study, okay?"

"Okay . . . reluctantly."

---

1. MANAGE CARB INTAKE TO REVERSE DIABETES

Foods containing carbs are quickly broken down by the digestive system into sugar, which enters the bloodstream and causes blood glucose levels to rise. That's why managing carbohydrate intake is key to defeating diabetes.

Not only does eating too many carbs increase blood sugar levels, it also over stimulates the release of insulin. Insulin doesn't just help cells use glucose; it signals the body to store extra calories as fat, which triggers weight gain!

Reducing total carb consumption is step one for weight loss and blood sugar control. The second step is making sure that, when he does eat carbs, he consumes the right ones.

Carbs Can Be Simple . . . or Complex

Simple carbs are sugars made of one or two sugar molecules. They're mostly empty calories and are bad for losing weight and fighting diabetes because they digest rapidly, leading to quick spikes in blood sugar and insulin levels . . . the absolute last thing someone trying to control diabetes needs! Simple carbohydrates are found in foods rich in white flour and added sugars—things like soda, cookies, sweetened cereals, white bread, white pretzels, and regular pasta.

In contrast, complex carbs are made of numerous sugar molecules strung together in a long chain. Complex carbs, or "good" carbs, are in their unrefined, "natural" state or close to it. They are found in foods like whole grains, beans and vegetables, and provide essential vitamins, minerals, and fiber. Because complex carb foods are packed with fiber they are digested slowly and help you feel full longer while providing sustained energy and stabilizing blood sugar levels.

Put simply: to help defeat diabetes he needs to limit the "bad" simple carbs like bagels, muffins, and candy and replace them with more "good" complex carbs like whole-grain products, beans, and vegetables.

Hubby Needs to Develop Strong Moral Fiber to Defeat Diabetes

When describing an upstanding person who is respected in their community, we often use the phrase, "He has strong moral fiber." Though many men may turn their nose up at the term, fiber is and always has been a positive word and a crucial weapon in helping to control diabetes and returning your husband to vibrant, youthful health.

As I said, fiber is a substance found in plants. Dietary fiber, the type of fiber we eat, has no calories and passes through the digestive system without being digested itself. There are two types of dietary fiber: soluble and insoluble. Both are important in maintaining health. Soluble fiber, which attracts water and turns into a gel when digested, helps to lower cholesterol levels. Insoluble provides bulk to the diet, which fills you up, and aids digestion.

To keep hubby satisfied and help him control his blood sugar levels, aim for meals that contain 10 to 15 grams of fiber. Most Americans only get about 15 grams per day. The Institute of Medicine recommends men consume about 38 grams per day and women about 25.

Fortunately, it's easy to find high-fiber foods. The number of grams of fiber per serving is listed right on the "Nutrition Facts" label of all packaged foods. When you shop for bread, cereals, pasta, and crackers, buy items that contain the most fiber per serving. For example, look for breads that contain at least 3 to 4 grams of fiber per slice and crackers that have at least 2 grams of fiber per serving. (Much more on translating food labels coming up next in chapter 7.)

Mike and Ellen's Top 10 Fiber Foods to Help Him Defeat Diabetes

1. **Split Peas:** 16 grams of fiber per cup, cooked. They're great in soups and stews.

2. **Lentils:** 16 grams fiber per cup, cooked. This quick-cooking bean is very versatile and can be used in soups, stews, and salads. Canned lentil soup makes a quick, simple lunch. Just heat it up, add a salad and some whole-grain crackers, and you're good to go! Shake in a few splashes of hot sauce if he likes things spicy.

3. **Black Beans:** 15 grams fiber per cup, cooked. Try premade black bean burgers (they're sold at Costco) for a quick lunch or dinner. (They're *good* . . . so sayeth carnivore Mike.)

4. **Bran Flakes:** 7 grams fiber per cup. Have a bowl for breakfast with low-fat milk, sprinkle them on yogurt, or use them to make high-fiber bran muffins.

5. **Oatmeal:** 4 grams fiber per cup, cooked. Add some fruit and milk for an easy morning meal.

6. **Whole-Wheat Pasta:** 4 grams fiber per cup, cooked. With a flavorful sauce he won't miss the white stuff. In fact, he probably won't notice at all.

7. **Raspberries:** 8 grams fiber per cup. Add them to cereal or yogurt. Buy frozen when they're not in season.

8. **Pears:** 5 grams fiber per medium fruit. They make great snacks and are delicious when caramelized. Michael loves them with pork chops. (Yes, he *can* have pork. Remember, it's about balance, not depravation.)

9. **Broccoli:** 2 grams fiber per cup. Fantastic as a stir-fry ingredient. Try dipping raw broccoli in hummus for a quick, energizing snack.

10. **Popcorn:** 3 cups popped have 3.5 grams of fiber. A great low-cal snack . . . as long as he skips the butter. (Feel free to use low-cal butter spray, or top the popcorn with powdered spices such as garlic, cumin, chili powder, or curry powder.) If he insists on eating while watching TV, this is your go-to snack for him.

Introduce fiber slowly. Too much fiber all at once when you're not used to it can leave some folks feeling bloated.

In the box, we've listed our top 10 favorite fiber foods to help your partner get a handle on his love handles and beat back diabetes. Include the ones he already likes in his meals and snacks, and experiment with some of the others to find more that he likes.

If your husband cries foul at the thought of replacing his pile of fries with a side of lentils, here are a few bonus tips to secretly increase his fiber intake:

- Add a little flaxseed meal to breading for chicken or fish.

- Purée cooked vegetables in the blender or food processor and add them to sauces, soups, and stews for a low-cal, high-fiber thickening.

- Use avocado (2 tablespoons contains 2 grams of fiber) as a sandwich spread instead of full-fat mayo.

Carb Counting: Easy As 1-2-3, Do-Re-Mi, A-B-C, Baby You and Me

Carbohydrate or "carb" counting—keeping track of how many grams of carbohydrates you eat per day—is a meal planning technique that can help him manage his blood sugar levels. The general recommendation from the American Diabetes Association is 45 to 60 grams of carbs for each meal. Snacks should contain between 15 and 30 grams of carbs.

Reading food labels (which we explain in detail in chapter 7) will tell you exactly how many carbs are in a serving of packaged foods.

One serving of starch contains 15 grams of carbs and 80 calories. In general, a single serving of starch equals:

- ½ cup of cooked cereal, or starchy vegetables such as potatoes
- ⅓ cup cooked rice
- 1 ounce of a bread product, about one slice
- ¾ to 1 ounce of most carbohydrate-based snack foods like crackers and chips

One serving of fruit contains 15 grams of carbs and 60 calories. In general a serving of fruit equals:

- ½ cup of fresh or unsweetened canned fruit
- 4 ounces of unsweetened fruit juice
- 1 medium piece of fresh fruit
- 2 tablespoons of dried fruit

One serving of low-fat milk (we do not recommend that people with prediabetes or type 2 diabetes drink full-fat milk) contains 12 grams of carbs and about 100 calories. In general one serving of milk equals:

- 1 cup of low-fat milk
- 6 ounces of low-fat yogurt

Counting carbs is important if you are taking insulin. If that is the case, you should speak with your doctor or health care team about your recommended carb intake. For the purposes of this book—which is focused on reversing type 2 diabetes so he doesn't have to take insulin and managing prediabetes so it doesn't become full-blown diabetes—carb counting is not required. Following our meal plan in chapter 12 and the healthy lifestyle changes we recommend should be enough to keep blood sugar in the healthy range. However, if hubby is an accountant who likes to count everything, he can certainly track his carbs.

Okay, so by controlling carbs, your partner has nailed the first "out" in his weight loss triple play. Here's the throw to second . . .

---

2. LEVERAGE HIS PROTEIN POWER

From hair and nails to bones, muscles, and blood, protein is a key component of every cell in our bodies. Protein is used to make hormones, enzymes, and other crucial body chemicals. Protein was named over 150 years ago after the Greek word *proteios*, meaning, "of prime importance."

Here's the good news about protein and diabetes:

- Many protein-rich foods like meat, poultry, eggs, and fish do not contain carbohydrates so they don't raise blood sugar levels.

- Eating protein stimulates the release of satiety hormones so your husband feels full and content longer.

- Eating protein and vegetables about 15 minutes before eating carbohydrates may help keep his blood sugar levels lower. A study showed that when people ate carbohydrates last (about 15 minutes after protein and vegetables), their blood sugar levels were about 29 percent lower after 30 minutes and 37 percent lower after 60 minutes!

However, don't overdo the protein. The average adult only needs 0.8 grams of protein per kilogram (about 2.2 pounds) of body weight. Two to three daily servings are all he needs. (For example, one serving of protein is a small steak, 4 ounces of canned tuna, or 1 cup of beans.) If he overdoes the protein, his body will just convert that extra protein into glucose if it's needed for energy or, worse, store it as fat.

To leverage his protein power, have him eat a small serving of protein at every meal and snack. (We're not talking fatty cold cuts or processed meats like bacon. Those are generally calorie bombs.) That's 2 to 5 ounces of lean meat such as three slices of lean roast beef, half a chicken breast, or a medium pork chop; 1 to 2 eggs; half a cup of fiber packed-beans; or 1 to 2 ounces of reduced-fat cheese. Fish, such as 4 ounces of tuna packed in water or 4 ounces of baked salmon, is always a great option because it's high in omega-3 fatty acids, which are good for his heart!

That's two outs! The man on third is heading for home. Here's the play at plate . . .

3. SELECT FAT SMARTLY

When it comes to fat, quantity and quality count. While protein and carbs have 4 calories per gram, fat has a whopping 9, so it's easy to overdo it.

It looks tempting to eliminate all fat from his diet as a way to lose weight, doesn't it? DON'T! Humans need to eat some fat to stay healthy. It just needs to be the right kind of fat.

The three broad categories of fat are saturated, trans, and

unsaturated (which includes monounsaturated fat and polyunsaturated fat). Although there's been quite a bit of debate recently about whether saturated fats are bad for you, numerous studies have shown that when you replace saturated fat with polyunsaturated fat, heart disease risk goes down. Saturated fats are not good for hubby because they increase LDL cholesterol levels (that's the "bad" cholesterol you've probably heard about; HDL is the "good" cholesterol), while unsaturated fats can help improve his cholesterol levels. Additional research has shown that reducing saturated fat may improve insulin sensitivity, which means lower blood sugar levels!

Saturated fats are usually solid at room temperature. They're found in foods such as margarine, full-fat dairy products (like regular cheeses and butter), and high-fat meats (like regular ground round, hot dogs, sausages, heavily marbled steaks and pork ribs). We say "usually" here, because even high-fat items such as whole milk—which obviously is not solid at room temperature—contain saturated fat.

We're not saying you must cut saturated fats out completely. Just use less and try to substitute healthier fats for the unhealthy ones. The American Heart Association recommends limiting saturated fats to no more than 7 percent of your calories, which is about 16 grams a day for someone on a 2,000-calorie diet. The best way to limit saturated fat is to eat fewer fatty animal products and to read labels. The grams of saturated fat as well as trans fat are always listed under "Nutrition Facts" on the labels of packaged foods.

Trans fats do not occur naturally. They are created in a food manufacturing process called hydrogenation that turns liquid fats into solids. (In fact, you can spot them in an ingredients list by looking for the word "hydrogenated.") They are usually found in fried and baked goods like pastries, crackers, and pie crust. STAY AWAY from trans fats as much as possible. They raise bad LDL cholesterol and lower the good HDL cholesterol.

Unsaturated fats are typically liquid at room temperature. They're found in foods like liquid vegetable oils (such as olive, canola, or safflower oil), but also in fish, avocados, nuts, and seeds. When used to replace saturated and trans fats, unsaturated fats can improve blood cholesterol levels, which may reduce your risk of heart disease and may benefit blood sugar control, which is especially helpful for type 2 diabetes. Healthy fats make food taste good, and like protein and fiber they help you feel full longer so you eat less.

The key is to use healthy fats to *replace* unhealthy fats. This is important. If you just *add* them to the diet, you'll be adding calories that hubby doesn't need. The American Heart Association recommends getting between 25 to 35 percent of your calories from fat, most of which should be unsaturated.

While you encourage your man to eat more healthy fats, you need to help him keep an eye on portion size. Half an ounce of peanuts (about 80 calories) or a tablespoon of peanut butter (90 calories) is a great snack. Half a cup of peanuts at 414 calories isn't going to help him lose weight. We suggest putting snack-size servings of nuts in individual plastic bags so he'll eat the perfect amount without going overboard.

Here are a few more suggestions to help him replace unhealthy fats with healthy ones:

- Eat 12 almonds instead of an ounce of cheese for a snack. The calories are about the same, but the almonds are healthier.

- Have a tablespoon of sunflower or pumpkin seeds as a salad topper instead of bacon or cheese.

- Use olive or canola oil to sauté foods instead of butter.

- Have a fish burger instead of a hamburger. (Salmon burgers are delicious! You'll find them in the frozen section of most grocery stores.)

- Try a tuna sandwich made with low-fat mayo instead of a salami and cheese sub.

And diabetes is out at home! That's the successful completion of your weight loss triple play!

Despite what you may have read elsewhere, there is no one ideal ratio of macronutrients: carbohydrates, protein, and fats. Calories come from all three. To help him lose weight and keep his blood sugar under control, you need to limit all three by making the "triple play" we describe in this chapter. The best advice is to help him make healthy food choices and teach him how to control his portion sizes. And remember: incorporate plenty of low-calorie, high-fiber plant foods with a little unsaturated fat to make his meals tasty and to keep him satisfied.

Chapter 7

Read It... Before He Eats it!
Food Label Literacy

One of the toughest challenges wives face when their husbands are diagnosed with diabetes is determining exactly what foods to buy. The average supermarket carries 42,214 food items. That's a lot to digest.

According to a Nielsen survey, nearly 59 percent of consumers have difficulty understanding nutrition labels. So step one in helping hubby get healthy starts before you even enter the store. You MUST learn to read food labels. Label knowledge will enable you to make quick, informed food choices that will help your husband lose weight, maintain normal blood sugar levels, unclog his arteries and keep his blood pressure low. Best of all . . . it's easy. Just follow our six-step food label fluency plan. Here it is:

FOOD LABELING: IT'S THE LAW!

All food manufacturers are required by law to reveal certain information about their products on a standardized food label, called "Nutrition Facts." When you know how to read one label, you know how to read them all. Yes, there are a few things food manufacturers try to hide, such as added sugars (which we'll explain how to uncover later in this chapter) and artificial ingredients. However, they must reveal serving size, calories, fat (total as well as saturated and trans fats), cholesterol, sodium (salt to us civilians), total carbohydrates (which includes fiber and sugar), protein, and certain vitamins and minerals.

Now, let's break it down . . .

OUR SIX-STEP FOOD LABEL FLUENCY PLAN

Take a look at this sample label:

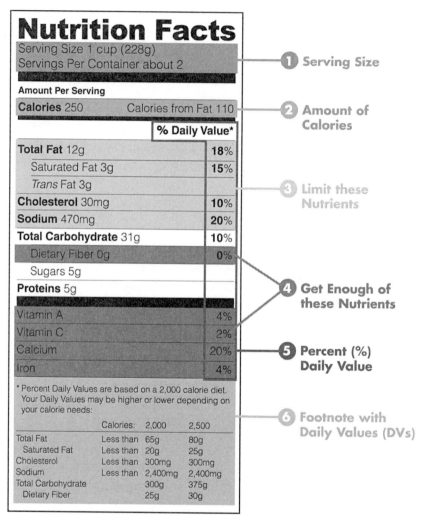

For educational purposes only. This label does not meet the labeling requirements described in 21 CFR 101.9.

The label is divided into six sections. The first five sections reveal specific information about the product itself. The sixth section is a footnote that provides general nutrition information. Once again, the format is the same on EVERY label.

Truth in Advertising

Ignore front-of-package health claims such as "cholesterol free," "fat free," "all natural," "no sugar added," "multigrain," or "made with whole grains." These are sales terms, not scientific descriptions. These marketing phrases have nothing to do with whether a food is healthy or not. To know that, you gotta read the Nutrition Facts label!

Section 1: Start Here

At the top of the label, right under "Nutrition Facts," you'll see both the serving size and the amount of servings per container. Paying attention to serving size is important for two reasons:

1. It determines all the other values listed on the label.
2. It tells you exactly how much ONE serving is. A serving for our sample label above (it's mac and cheese, by the way) is 1 cup, and the package contains 2 servings. One serving is fine for a light meal or side dish. The whole box? Tooooo much.

"I Can't Believe I Ate the Whole Thing"

Tip: Gently remind hubby that unless the label lists "Servings Per Container" as "1" the entire package is *not* a serving. To help him cut down on calories, encourage him to measure out *one* serving. His new mantra: *A box is not a serving . . . A box is not a serving . . . A box is not a serving . . .*

Serving size is listed in familiar amounts such as cups or pieces, followed by the metric weight (i.e., the number of grams). Serving size is supposed to represent how much of a certain food an "average person" would consume at a meal or snack. (Clearly the label makers haven't seen teens eat.) They are usually standardized to ensure that different products in the same food category have the same or similar serving sizes. For example, a serving of milk—whether whole, 2%, 1%, skim, strawberry, or chocolate—is always 1 cup. This makes it easy to compare similar food items to determine what's healthier for hubby. In our milk example, you'd quickly be able to tell from the label that skim milk is lower in fat, calories, and sugar than strawberry or chocolate milk and clearly the healthier choice.

Section 2: Check Calories

Right under serving size, you'll see "Calories." This tells you how many calories are in *one* serving (again, not the whole package; just one serving) as well as how many of those calories come from fat. Pay attention to calories per serving! When choosing food items where there are a ton of options, such as cereals or salad dressings, pick the product with the fewest calories.

Section 3: Limit These Nutrients

Section 3 lists nutrients that most people get too much of anyway and should limit because they can increase your risk of certain chronic diseases (like heart disease), some cancers, and high blood pressure. These nutrients include total fat, saturated fat, cholesterol, and sodium.

✓ *The skinny on fat.* Fat is high in calories (9 calories per gram versus protein and carbohydrates, which have 4), so selecting lower-fat items can help him eat fewer calories and lose weight. Look for items low in saturated fat and trans fat. These fats are associated with increased LDL (again, bad) cholesterol levels and risk of heart and blood vessel diseases, both common diabetes complications. He should limit them.

✓ *Cholesterol confusion.* Let's take a moment to clear up some confusion about cholesterol. The conventional wisdom used to be that foods such as red meat and eggs were bad for you because they contributed to cholesterol buildup. But that mixes up two broad types of cholesterol. No, not LDL and HDL—here we're talking about *dietary* cholesterol and *blood* cholesterol.

Dietary and blood cholesterol are not the same thing. Dietary cholesterol is found in animal products such as eggs, shrimp, and red meat. Blood (also called serum) cholesterol is a waxy, fat-like substance found in the body's cells. People with high cholesterol levels (especially bad LDL cholesterol, which causes a buildup of cholesterol in your arteries) have a greater risk of heart disease.

While previously the Dietary Guidelines for Americans recommended limiting cholesterol intake to 300 milligrams a day, that recommendation has changed. Cholesterol is no longer a nutrient of concern because new evidence shows that dietary cholesterol doesn't have a major negative impact on blood cholesterol. So shrimp and eggs are back on his menu.

✓ *Pass (on) the salt, please.* Remember to look for foods low in sodium. Too much sodium can elevate blood pressure. Most people with diabetes develop high blood pressure during their life, and high blood pressure can trigger or worsen diabetes complications, including eye and kidney diseases. Adults who need to lower their blood pressure should limit sodium to 2,400 milligrams a day (that's about a teaspoonful). Below 1,500 is even better.

✓ *Those pesky carbs again.* For diabetics it's important to look at the "Total Carbohydrate" line, which includes all sugars, complex carbohydrates, and fiber. THIS NUMBER IS VERY IMPORTANT, because all types of carbs can influence blood glucose levels. Review the steps we listed in chapter 6 to manage your husband's carbohydrate intake.

Section 4: Get Enough of These Nutrients

Next on the label are important nutrients that Americans don't get enough of in their diet, including dietary fiber, vitamins A and C, calcium, and iron. (Although protein is also listed in this section, most Americans already get plenty in their normal diets.) Eating these nutrients improves health and reduces the risk of some diseases. For example, getting enough calcium reduces your risk of the bone disease osteoporosis.

To reverse diabetes as well as reduce blood cholesterol levels, it's particularly important to make sure he's eating plenty of dietary fiber. Fiber is good for him because it slows down digestion and helps keep blood sugar levels stable. Fiber will also fill him up so he'll eat less. To help him get at least 38 grams of fiber per day (the recommendation for men), look for foods high in fiber. Hint: Select grain products (such as crackers, bread, pasta, or cereal) that contain at least 3 grams of fiber (the more the better) per serving. And don't forget our list of top 10 favorite fiber foods in chapter 6!

Section 5: Percent Daily Values (%DV)

These numbers are listed on the right side of the label next to the nutrients you want to limit or get enough of. This number, which is based on the recommended amount a person on a 2,000-calorie diet should eat, will help you determine if a serving of this food is relatively high or low in that nutrient. A figure of 5 percent or less is considered low, and 20 percent or more is considered high. For example, the food for our sample label is high in sodium (which is bad) and calcium (which is good) and low in fiber, vitamins A and C, and iron, all of which you want to eat more of.

Section 6: Footnote

Section 6 is a footnote explaining the "Percent Daily Values" based on a 2,000-calorie diet. Some labels (it's not required) also include general nutrition information that provides upper limits for total fat, saturated fat, cholesterol, and sodium and lower limits for total carbohydrate and fiber that an average person who's consuming either 2,000 or 2,500 calories per day should eat.

DECIPHERING THE INGREDIENT LIST

Understanding the ingredient list and what it can tell you about the foods your husband consumes can really help him (and you) turbocharge his diet with tasty, diabetes-defeating fare. The list is usually next to or under the Nutrition Facts label, but you may find it elsewhere on the package.

> **Ingredients:** Whole grain wheat, raisins, wheat bran, sugar, brown sugar syrup, contains 2% or less of salt, malt flavor.
> **Vitamins and Minerals:** Potassium chloride, niacinamide, reduced iron, vitamin B_6 (pyridoxine hydrochloride), zinc oxide, vitamin B_2 (riboflavin), vitamin B_1 (thiamin hydrochloride), vitamin A palmitate, folic acid, vitamin D_3, vitamin B_{12}.
> **CONTAINS WHEAT INGREDIENTS.**

Manufacturers must list all the ingredients in order of volume. In other words, the ingredient listed first on the list (and second, third, and so on) is present in greater amounts than the ingredients that are listed after it. For the purpose of this book, we are going to focus on the ingredient list items that affect diabetes the most: whole grains and added sugars. However there are a few other unhealthy food ingredients that you want to avoid:

- Try to steer clear of sodium nitrite and sodium nitrate, two preservatives in some processed luncheon meats (like baloney and salami) that may pose a cancer risk.

- Remember, any ingredient containing the word "sodium" just means added salt.

- Don't buy products that contain partially hydrogenated oils, which are a common source of unhealthy trans fats.

Whole Grains

To identify fiber-rich foods, look for the word "whole" before the name of a grain: whole wheat, whole grain wheat, whole grain wheat flour, or whole grain rye flour. (Popcorn, oatmeal, and quinoa are also considered whole grains.) When you buy products such as breakfast cereals, pasta, breads, and crackers, make sure the word "whole grain" or some equivalent appears as the first or second ingredient. Don't be fooled by such healthy-sounding ingredients as "unbleached enriched flour" as the first ingredient—it's not the same as whole grain.

Sugar

The United States Department of Agriculture (USDA) recommends that Americans limit their intake of foods and drinks with added sugar to less than 10 percent of their daily calorie intake. That's about 50 grams, 200 calories, or 12 teaspoons per day. The American Heart Association recommends no more than 100 calories per day (about 6 teaspoons) for women and no more than 150 calories per day (about 9 teaspoons) for men. That's not a lot when you consider that a 12-ounce can of Coca-Cola contains 39 grams of sugar and a Chocolate Fudge Pop-Tart contains 20 grams.

Currently there is no way to tell exactly how much sugar has been added to a food. Food manufacturers do not have to reveal how much sugar they *add* to foods, just the total amount of sugar that's in the foods. The word "Sugar" that you see under "Total Carbohydrates" on the Nutrition Facts label includes both natural sources (like the sugars found in fruit and dairy products) as well as added sugars used to sweeten foods.

Food manufacturers are sneaky. They use multiple names for sugar in the ingredients list and several types of sugar in one product so sweeteners appear further down the list . . . fooling you into thinking there isn't much sugar in their product after all. Common ingredient list names for sugar include sugar, cane sugar, evaporated cane juice, molasses, honey, malted barley extract, corn syrup, corn sweetener, fructose, high fructose corn syrup, fruit juice concentrate, glucose, malt syrup, dextrose, sucrose, and lactose. To avoid added sugar, buy packaged foods that contain NO sugar or at least don't have any type of sweetener listed as one of the first five ingredients.

Remember, *there is NO SUCH THING as a healthy added sugar*, especially for diabetics. Studies have linked added sugar with weight gain, obesity, decreased consumption of essential nutrients, and increased risk of heart disease. Added sugars are quickly broken down by the digestive system, converted to glucose, and dumped into the bloodstream. The sweet stuff causes insulin and blood sugar levels to spike, exactly what you don't want to happen with diabetes.

All sugars react in your body the same. Whether some marketer calls their sugar "natural" or "organic," it's still sugar. Agave sugar is still sugar—just like the sugar on your table—that you'll take away so he doesn't add it to his Frosted Flakes, which should disappear too. They all make his blood sugar go up, up, up.

The bottom line: your man doesn't have to cut out sugar entirely, but he must limit how much sugar he eats, regardless of the source. While enjoying the occasional sweet treat such as a couple of cookies or a scoop of ice cream is fine, you want to make sure to keep hidden sugar from sneaking into his bloodstream, undermining all the hard work the two of you are doing to get and keep him healthy.

Artificial Sweeteners Are Not the Answer

While artificial sweeteners may seem like a diabetic solution and calorie bargain, they are associated with weight gain, not loss. Research shows people who drank diet soda gained almost four times as much belly fat over nine years as those who didn't drink diet soda. Another study found women who drank one 20-ounce diet soda per day had a 66 percent increased risk of diabetes! Diet sodas are so intensely sweet they can alter your taste buds so you crave sweeter and sweeter foods. Studies show that artificial sweeteners disrupt normal biological signals that control hunger and satiety, resulting in overeating. So take it from us: substituting artificial sweetener for sugar is *not* the same as cutting back on sugar!

Now that you're an expert in food label interpretation let's take your new knowledge out for a spin and go shopping.

Chapter 8

Food Planning and Shopping the Feng Shui Way

Feng shui is a Chinese philosophical system of harmonizing one-self with the surrounding environment. Feng shui (pronounced *fung shway*) can be applied to health, marriage, money . . . and your refrigerator. By "feng shui-ing" your shopping, we mean bringing the foods you buy and use into harmony with the necessity of defeating diabetes . . . now!

In this chapter we are going to tell you how to plan meals and snacks, what to buy, and especially what *not* to buy to keep hubby healthy. We will also incorporate info from the previous chapters to build his new, diabetes-defeating nutritional profile. Yes, we've done all the work for you. Now, let's take the information and techniques we've been discussing and apply them to his plate and waistline as we feng shui your refrigerator.

BUILDING THE BALANCED MEAL PLAN

Healthy diabetes-defeating meals don't just happen! You need to plan, shop, and prepare. Yes, it takes extra work. But it's a bit of work that can make the difference between a long, healthy, happy life together or a short, painful future filled with diabetic complications—with *you* being his 24/7 nurse. You don't want that and neither does he. Remember, if the right foods are available (and the wrong foods aren't), he'll eat the right things.

The key to creating healthy meals is PLANNING. Planning saves time, money, and calories. A little effort goes a long way when it comes to defeating diabetes, and this is where you can have a big impact on his health with minimal effort.

Men love to plan and feel like they're in charge. (Silly things, aren't they?) So make him part of the feng shui planning! Sit down and discuss what meals the two of you will be eating that week. Start out with dinner since it requires the most planning. (Breakfast and lunch remain somewhat similar from day to day.) Of course, when he insists on buying a large nacho chip pie with heavy cream frosting, you're gonna have to talk him down into a more reasonable snack. When this happens, take a soothing approach and ask him, "You want to die, sucker?"

Feng Shui Step 1: Planning

The first feng shui step is to plan with hubby as we discussed above. See, you've already used feng shui . . . wasn't that easy? When planning his diet the feng shui way, keep three principles in mind: variety, balance, and moderation.

✓ *Variety* entails choosing different foods both across and within food groups. The point is to mix it up and try new, healthy foods. Don't just buy bananas and iceberg lettuce; throw a mango and some cauliflower into the cart. Try garlic-infused multigrain crackers or higher fiber blue corn chips instead of yellow. Is he a meat man? Try buffalo burger. Available in most supermarkets, buffalo tastes great and is an excellent source of low-fat, low-cal protein. Variety will help you keep healthy, diabetes-defeating meals interesting, which is really important. You don't want him to start eating his old diabetes-inflaming diet again out of boredom.

✓ *Balance* is key to keeping him satisfied and properly nourished while he loses weight. You need to balance the type and amount of foods he eats during each meal, as well as throughout the day and week. To build balance, serve him a combination of protein foods, dairy, whole grains, and produce.

✓ *Moderation* means having him eat the foods he likes while keeping portions under control so he can reach and maintain a healthy weight. In other words, don't overdo any food. For example, if he's at a party and cake and cookies are served, moderation means choosing a small slice of cake or a cookie or two (depending on size), not both. At the buffet table, moderation means having one fried appetizer and then filling (not overfilling) his plate with healthy options such as cocktail shrimp, salad, and fruit.

Buffet Buffers

Does your partner love those all-you-can-eat buffets? While we don't recommend making them a weekly affair, he can enjoy them occasionally. Here are some tips based on research conducted at the Food and Brand Lab at Cornell University.

✓ Sit further away. For every 40 feet further away from the serving area, people make one less trip to the buffet.

✓ Got your back. Have him sit with his back to the buffet so he can't see the food.

✓ Be selective. Before he fills his plate, teach him to look over all the options, then choose the one or two items he really wants.

To help you plan his meals and incorporate all his essential macronutrients (carbs, fat, and protein) and food groups (grains, fruits, vegetables, dairy and meats), we've created a complete Diabetes-Defeating Meal Plan for him (so you don't have to!) in chapter 12. The plan is also a nifty tool to help him track what he's eaten. Remember chapter 5? Self-monitoring and food tracking *will* help him lose weight!

After planning his meals and snacks, make a healthy shopping list. Guess what? To help you get started, later in this chapter we're going to tell you exactly what to buy. No thanks necessary, it's just how we roll. But this is important: When you head to the store, do not skip the list! Without a list, people often buy items they had no intention of purchasing. Supermarkets encourage and rely on this type of behavior. They literally set booby traps (chips, soda, and cookies at the end of the aisles and candy at the checkout line) to get you to buy foods you and hubby do not need.

Prior to feng shui-ing your food shopping, make sure you

practice reading food labels at home. Building your label-reading skills will make it easer for you to use nutrition labels to make quick, informed food choices that will help defeat diabetes.

Feng Shui Step 2: Shopping

Your second feng shui step is to shop without hubby. He will just mess up the feng shui by putting tater tots, breaded cheese balls, and pie in your cart. Instead of enjoying a harmonious shopping experience, you'll be arguing with him about what to buy, which creates friction (the point of feng shui is to erase friction and create harmony). When his taste buds have adapted to his new diet, then it's safe to shop with him. There's nothing wrong with buying the occasional fun-sized treat, but you don't want to bring a boatload of junk food into the house. Those days are over! Remember, the behavior chain in chapter 5? To break the chain, *do not let massive amounts of junk food over the threshold.* Remember, the best way to help a junk food junkie is to "just say no!"

Feng Shui Step 3: Staying On Course

The third and final feng shui step is to stay on course when you enter the supermarket. Stick to your list of healthy food choices. (Important tip: hunger reduces willpower and makes controlled shopping difficult. So don't shop on an empty stomach.) The healthiest items in most grocery stores tend to be on the perimeter of the store. This is where you'll find the products he needs to defeat diabetes: fresh fruits, vegetables, low-fat dairy products, and lean meats.

Now, grab your cart and let's get started . . .

■ Produce the Goods

Start in the produce section, which is typically near the entrance just past the flowers. Other than starchy vegetables like potatoes, winter squash, and corn, produce is very low in calories and great for your mate. Most veggies have around 25 calories per serving (½ cup cooked or 1 cup raw) and fruit has around 60 calories per serving (1 medium piece or ½ cup). So buy plenty of produce—it will help him lose weight by filling him up without filling him out.

Buy a variety of produce, meaning different types with different colors. Colors reflect different vitamins, minerals, and phytochemicals (plant chemicals) found in each fruit or vegetable. Research suggests that foods high in phytochemicals may directly help reverse diabetes, most likely by reducing inflammation and increasing insulin sensitivity. Eating brightly colored fruits and veggies also helps ensure that he's getting plenty of protective, healthy nutrients. Tip: usually, the darker the color of a fruit or vegetable, the higher the nutrient content.

Buy three or more types of fruits and four or more types of veggies. We always stock apples and bananas (great for snacks and smoothies) and one or two other types of fruit, usually what's on sale and/or in season.

We buy one type of lettuce, a dark leafy green like spinach to cook with, plus three or four additional veggies such as carrots, celery, or broccoli.

Next, throw a bag of potatoes in the cart. Sure they're starchy, but a medium russet is very filling, only contains about 168 calories and 37 grams of carbs, and is a great platform for additional veggies like sautéed spinach with a sprinkling of Parmesan cheese. Just don't let him turn his potato into a diabetic calorie bomb by larding on the butter, sour cream, or cheese. Sweet potatoes are a great option because the complex carbohydrates they contain are converted to blood sugar more slowly than the carbs in white potatoes.

Retailers put older produce items on top and in front, so reach back and dig down for the freshest items. (This is also true with dairy products, eggs, and meat.) Try to buy produce during the week, as it's typically delivered Monday through Friday.

Frozen produce is a great option to add quick nutrition to meals and snacks. Stocking frozen produce automatically feng shui's your fridge because it crowds out unhealthy items that you may have stocked previously, such as ice cream, French fries, and frozen pizza. We always stock Asian frozen vegetables for quick stir-fries, frozen green beans for an easy side dish, and frozen spinach for all sorts of cooking. Adding a handful of veggies to sauces and soups is a great way to make them more nutritious, increase volume healthfully, and lower the number of calories per serving. We also stock frozen berries for snacking, to add to smoothies, yogurt, and cereal, and to throw at the dog. (Don't do this if you have a long-haired dog. The berries will get stuck in her coat.)

While you're in the produce aisle, pick up some vegetarian "meat" products. These low-fat, soy-based cold cuts are healthy, great in sandwiches, and save calories. Plus, research shows eating soy may help him lower his cholesterol level. Also, grab some tofu (it's usually stocked there) for stir-fries.

We know what you're thinking: there's no way my guy is going to eat tofu. Chances are, he's probably been enjoying tofu all his life at Chinese restaurants without noticing it. Tofu pops up in fried rice, stir-fries, stews, and many other Asian dishes. Sure, tofu can be bland. That's why in chapter 12, Mike and Ellen's Diabetes-Defeating Meal Plan, we're going to show you how to spice it up so he'll love it.

■ Show Me the Bread

After produce, you'll typically find the bakery section. This section's wonderful smells and tempting treats are designed to make you feel hungry (see the salivating zombies caressing cupcakes, frosted donuts and crunchy rolls?), so avert your eyes and walk on by . . . quickly. Bypassing the cupcakes, donuts, and crunchy rolls is a no-brainer, but the extra-large muffins (even if they're bran) and fresh-baked French bread (made with white flour)? Forgetaboutit! Stay focused, stick to your list, and buy what's good for hubby.

In the regular bread aisle, look for products that are as complex as possible. (Remember simple carbs versus complex carbs?) Pick up a loaf of whole-grain high-fiber bread, a package of whole-grain English muffins, and either whole-grain pita bread or flat bread. Again, don't be fooled by the name on the package or the color of the bread. For example, rye and pumpernickel may look and sound like they're whole grain, but they aren't.

Checking off the rest of the carb items on your shopping list, you'll also want to purchase a few boxes of whole-grain pasta and a bag of brown rice for healthy side dishes.

■ Meat Up

Think lean and you won't have to be mean at dinner. Buy lean cuts of beef (flank, sirloin, and tenderloin), pork (tenderloin, well-trimmed chops, or roast), ground turkey breast, and chicken. Don't forget to check out the seafood section. Fish and shellfish are naturally low in fat and calories. However, avoid fresh or frozen seafood with added breading such as fish sticks, which can be high in calories. Canned tuna and sardines packed in water (not oil) are great items to keep in your pantry for quick, energetic meals and snacks.

Remember earlier when we told you to cut out the cold cuts? If hubby just has to have 'em, then pick up some lean ones (such as turkey breast, ham, Canadian bacon, or lean roast beef) for quick sandwiches. Just go easy on the mayo, and stuff those sandwiches with fresh greens, tomatoes, and other nutritious low calorie options.

■ Can It

Venture into the canned food aisle and stock up on beans, a powerful diabetes-defeating food packed with fiber. We suggest keeping chickpeas (great in salads), white beans (soups and pasta), kidney beans (minestrone) and refried beans (great in Mexican dishes and dips) in the pantry. Although the name "refried" implies they are high in fat, there are plenty of low fat varieties available. That's why we taught you how to read labels in the previous chapter!

■ Nuts to You

Pick up one or two kinds of nuts (unsalted if he has blood pressure issues) such as almonds or peanuts. High in protein and healthy fat, they're a smart snack (much better than chips) that won't wreak havoc on his blood sugar level. Just make sure he only eats about an ounce (the amount that will fit in the palm of your hand or a shot glass), because they are relatively high in calories. Almonds are a great choice because they're the lowest in calories. A single ounce of almonds is about 23 nuts.

▪ Milk It

Don't forget dairy products, which are a great source of protein. The key with dairy is to buy fat-free or low-fat products. These include skim or 1% milk, low-fat or fat-free unsweetened yogurt, and low-fat cheeses often labeled as "part skim," "reduced-fat," or "fat-free." Remember, milk and yogurt contain carbs. Just 1 cup of milk or 6 ounces of plain nonfat yogurt has 12 grams of carbohydrates, so you have to help him keep track of them in his meal plan.

▪ Eggceptional

You'll also want to buy eggs, which are packed with protein and great for quick meals. (We always keep several hard-boiled eggs in the fridge for satisfying snacks.) As we mentioned in chapter 7, researchers used to think eating foods high in dietary cholesterol, like eggs, raised blood cholesterol levels. However, according to the latest US government findings, dietary cholesterol now is "not considered a nutrient of concern for overconsumption" because the latest scientific evidence "shows no appreciable relationship" between heart disease and how much cholesterol you eat. It's the saturated fat and trans fats that you need to limit to reduce his blood cholesterol levels and lower his risk of heart disease and stroke. So . . . eggs are okay.

▪ Snack Attack

Snacks are definitely part of his meal plan, so buy him healthy versions of his favorite munchies. Look for and buy two or three types of crackers, pretzels, or corn chips that contain at least 3 grams of fiber per serving. Remember, just because they're healthier doesn't mean he can eat the whole bag. Check out how large a serving size is and give him just a bit under that. When he groans, give him a few more, up to the suggested serving size. Yes, it is manipulative. Yes, it works.

▪ The Cereal Bowl

When he's rushed in the morning, a bowl of cereal with low-fat milk may be all he has time for. Fortunately, there are lots of high-fiber, low-sugar, diabetic-friendly options. Smack him if he asks for Honey Smacks—one cup has more sugar than a Twinkie! Skip the Captain Crunch (44 percent sugar!), Fruit Loops with Fruity Shaped Marshmallows (48 percent sugar!), and Sugar Frosted Flakes, which contains 11 grams of sugar. Tony the Tiger had to retire recently due to diabetic complications.

Feng shui-ing is about balance. So balance what he *needs* to eat to defeat diabetes with the items he *likes* to eat so he's not tempted to call Domino's behind your back. Follow our shopping plan and you're off to a great start of healthy, diabetes-defeating eating.

Chapter 9

Eating Right When He's Eating Out

When diabetes enters the picture, a lot of folks think eating out is ... well, out. Wrong! Your favorite restaurant is still a safe, happy destination. (Unless of course it's Freddy's Fried Dough Emporium. In which case hubby needs to find a new favorite.) Fortunately, nowadays most restaurants (especially chains) have healthy meal options and are willing to work with customers to make sure you enjoy yourself.

A NIGHT ON THE TOWN: PLAYING IT FUN AND SMART

When eating out, let him get whatever he wants, but within reason. Don't be the "food nanny," monitoring every bite. Have fun! Isn't that the point of eating out? Why order an overpriced, wilting salad when he really wants steak? To compensate, cut down a bit before or after your night out.

Unlike what a lot of doctors tell you, it's okay to have fun when you're a diabetic. In fact, it's essential to your health! Having fun with your food actually results in eating less and enjoying it more. When you eat *mindfully*, you take the time to savor every bite and use all your senses to fully experience the pleasures of eating. When you're paying restaurant prices, it makes a lot of sense to slowwww-www down and enjoyyyyyyyyy every ... single ... bite.

Now we're going to show you how to find the hidden fat and calories on a menu so he will know what he's *really* consuming ... and how to avoid them. This information will allow the two of you to control his fat and calorie intake. He'll *know* what he's putting into his body and the effect it will have on his blood sugar.

The first order of business: learn menu lingo to uncover hidden blood sugar bombs:

- *Crispy* means deep-fried.

- *Topped with* or *Covered in* usually means extra calories from things like cream sauces, cheese, or sour cream.

- *Au gratin* refers to a dish that is baked with a topping of bread crumbs and cheese . . . lots of cheese.

- *Battered* is a good description of what his blood sugar will be like after eating foods dredged in flour, eggs, and bread crumbs and then deep-fried. Does he just love battered shrimp? Here's an easy solution: trade battered for cocktail shrimp or shrimp broiled with a little garlic butter. By cutting out all the other dia-betes-*increasing* elements, he can enjoy the indulgence of but-tery shrimp without guilt.

- *Basted* usually means meat swimming in sauces sweetened with high-fructose corn syrup, molasses, or other sugars.

- *Barbecue* . . .

"Stop right there, Ellen. Now you've gone too far. Barbecue is sacrosanct!"

"Sorry, Michael, you make world-class Q at home but when eating out, barbecue usually means fatty meat swimming in sauces super high in sugar."

"Okay, as long as you're not talking about my lean and mean black pepper–encrusted smoked ribs, I'll let it slide . . . this time. Nobody messes with my Q!"

- *Creamed*, when associated with vegetables, usually means thick, buttery, or cream-based sauces that overwhelm the nutritional benefits veggies have.

- *Stuffed* anything is usually made with lots of bread or bread crumbs to add heft to the oyster, cheese, bacon, pasta, or other food being "stuffed." Generally high in white carbs and fat.

- *Flash-fried, wok-fried, skillet-fried, pan-fried*—all mean the same thing: fried, fried, fried.

- *Fried rice.* Do we really have to say it?

- *Tempura* is a Japanese word meaning fried seafood or fried vegetables.

FLYING SOLO

What about the times when you are not around to help hubby decipher the diabetic red flags on restaurant menus? When he's out with his buddies, he's just going to have to show some discipline. Nachos and bottomless beer during the NCAA basketball playoffs may be sacred to him, but now he needs to find healthier ways to hang out with the boys. A good start is to eat a light, healthy meal before he even goes out so he can resist gorging himself on the mountains of sour cream, cheese sauce and diabetes inflaming chips his buddies order. He can also order his own light beers (approximately half the carbs of regular beer). Many sports bars now serve healthy options as well. If he can't resist, try ordering a grilled chicken salad, cocktail shrimp, or a broth-based soup. We're talking minestrone soup here, not cream- and butter-rich clam chowder!

Work-related meals can be another challenge. But they don't have to be. Treat business meals like business. He's not there for fun; he's there to accomplish a goal. Focus on the goal, not the food. When working, he should order light to stay sharp. Let the client indulge. Focus on showing them a good time, not on the food. Gorging himself in front of clients sends the wrong message anyway. Again, it's another situation where he has to show discipline. Get the account and have his fun later.

An Old, Very Effective, Portion-Control Trick

Don't be afraid to ask for a doggie bag. The rest of that T-bone is still going to taste great for a fun meal tomorrow. The double-fried potatoes with butter-basted grits, cheese sauce, and bacon biscuits . . . *"No thanks. We'll leave those."*

For the man who travels a lot, ordering food from the hotel kitchen (especially if his employer is picking up the tab) is often a healthy, great-tasting option. They can pack a healthy breakfast, sandwich, or salad for lunch so Sammy's Sloppy Sub Shop won't tempt him when he gets hungry. The hotel wants to please, so they'll get him what he needs.

ETHNIC IS OFTEN A HEALTHY OPTION

Whether on the road or out on the town with you, as a diabetic he has to be choosier about the types of restaurants he frequents. Buffets and barbecue pits (sorry, Michael) should be low on the list. Fortunately, our country is blessed with eateries from every imaginable corner of the globe, and they all offer delicious options for the health-conscious guest. Here are some of our favorites . . .

Asian

Asian cuisines are a fantastic option due to the abundance of vegetables, seafood, and cooking methods that use little or no oil, tempura being one of the exceptions. For example, Vietnamese cuisine relies less on frying and heavy sauces and tends to use water or broth instead of oils. Chinese stir-fries can also be a great option because they are cooked in very little oil and usually include plenty of healthy veggies, especially broccoli and greens like nutrient-rich bok choy. (We're talking about decent restaurants here, not all-you-can-eat buffets or greasy chow mein delivery joints with health inspection certificates in the window from 1982.) Asian cuisines are also rich in soy (think tofu, edamame, and miso), which is a great source of low-calorie protein. When eating Asian, try to swap the white rice for brown. Too much white rice can spike blood sugar levels. Many restaurants serve brown rice, and some even make sushi with brown rice.

While Japanese cuisine includes some fried dishes, it also features broth-based dishes and utilizes the stir-fry method. In Japan they have a practice called *hara hachi bu*. Yep, it sounds like something you'd say on Halloween, but it means, "Eat until you are 80 percent full." Nothing scary about that! Following this simple rule will make a big difference in your husband's waistline in just a few of months.

He can eat regular sushi in moderation occasionally. Stick to 6 to 12 pieces and stay away from sushi made with tempura, which is fried and high in fat and calories. Good choices include a California roll (about 46 calories per piece, 6 grams of carbs), avocado roll (about 41 calories per piece, 6 grams carbs), spicy tuna roll (about 48 calories per piece, 4 grams carbs), cucumber roll (about 23 calories per piece, 5 grams carbs), or tuna nigiri (two pieces over rice have 106 calories and 17 grams carbs including the rice). Another good option is sashimi, which is just the raw fish without rice and is very low in calories and virtually carb-free! Seaweed salad is also a great choice . . .

"Ellen, stop! You're getting carried away. Men aren't going to order seaweed salad. I bet women reading this right now are saying, 'Seaweed? Not my Harry.'"

"But I love seaweed salad."

"Ellen . . . We need to move on."

"Okay, forget it. More seaweed for me."

Mediterranean

Mediterranean cuisine developed in countries adjacent to the Mediterranean Sea, including Greece, Southern Italy, Portugal, and parts of Spain. According to research conducted by Harvard University, the Mediterranean diet is linked to slower aging and is associated with significantly less risk of death from heart disease and cancer.

People tend to lose weight and feel more satisfied on this diet. It's filled with healthy fats, fresh fruits and vegetables (at least 6 to 7 servings per day), high-fiber beans, whole grains, and omega-3–rich fish, all of which are immune-boosting and diabetes-fighting ingredients. Remember, go easy on the pasta and make it whole wheat. Stick to about 1 cup cooked pasta per meal. Skip appetizers such as spanakopita (those yummy spinach and feta cheese pastries you get at Greek restaurants) that are made with lots of butter.

Indian

Indian cuisine is filled with healthy, flavorful spices, many of which have healing properties. Indian cuisine also contains yogurt, which research suggests helps fight diabetes, as well as fiber-rich lentils (found in the traditional Indian dish dal), which can help stabilize blood sugar. Good choices include tandoori roti, fiber-rich whole-grain bread that's more diabetic-friendly than refined Indian breads like chapati and dosa. Chana masala is a flavorful chickpea-based dish packed with fiber. Vegetable curry contains a variety of nutrient-dense veggies like eggplant, spinach, and carrots. Bhindi, a flavorful Indian side dish, contains the vegetable okra. One study found that eating a serving of okra a day for six months improved kidney health in diabetics. Avoid fried appetizers such as samosas and curries made with cream and butter. Keep servings of bread and rice to a minimum.

Mexican

We know what you're thinking: nacho platters loaded with fried chips, cheese, and sour cream with a pile of chimichangas (basically a deep-fried burrito) on the side. Hubby love him some Mex? Then try the light, healthy side of Mexican cuisine. That means fresh salsa, beans (black or pinto), brown rice, soup (black bean or gazpacho), and enchiladas made with low-fat cheese and beans or chicken. Or try our favorite, make-at-home healthy fajitas. Just stir-fry marinated chicken strips or shrimp with peppers and onions, serve in a whole-grain flour tortilla or corn tortilla, add some salsa and you've got a quick, simple, tasty dinner that'll make him say "Olé!"

FAST FOOD ISN'T OFF THE MENU

They don't call the USA "Fast Food Nation" for nothin'! According to various sources, there are currently almost a quarter million fast food outlets in the United States. That's a lot of opportunities to tempt your husband with double meat subs, pepperoni slices, and diabetic catastrophes like chicken fried steak with bacon gravy and buttermilk cheddar biscuits. And he doesn't even have to get out of the car and walk 30 feet across a parking lot to get it—just drive up, order up, and his blood sugar goes up, up, up!

But here's the surprising thing: fast food can actually be a good choice, especially when he's on the road. The key is education so he knows what he's ordering before he gets to the drive-thru window. A decade ago, if you pulled off the highway for a fast-food lunch or dinner, your only healthful options were either a wilted salad made with iceberg lettuce and a few carrot bits or a cardboard chicken sandwich. Today, fast food offers many healthy options loaded with fresh ingredients. Here are a few healthful options for the diabetic road warrior:

- ✓ *McDonalds:* Grilled chicken sandwich (skip the mayo and it weighs in at 300 calories) or Mexican-style salad with grilled chicken, fruit, and walnuts on the side.

- ✓ *Burger King:* Have a Whopper Jr. (skip the mayo) with a side salad. Go ahead and order it with cheese and you're still at only around 350 calories. We hope we no longer have to say this but . . . ixnay on the fries.

- ✓ *Wendy's:* Our favorite pick is chili. It's only 250 calories (without crackers or cheese), high in protein, and contains 5 grams of fiber.

- ✓ *Subway:* A six-inch Turkey Breast Sandwich (ask for extra veggies) on nine-grain bread makes for a satisfying meal for only around 280 calories.

Fast food restaurants are required to have nutrition information about their food posted on the premises. They often list calories on the menu board right next to the price. In addition, detailed nutrition info is usually listed on the company websites. Just Google the name of the restaurant and "nutrition information." Or check out www.fastfoodnutrition.org.

See, eating right when you're eating out isn't really that hard. So let him go ahead and enjoy . . . just not *too* much. ☺

Chapter 10

All The Right Moves
Your Personal Road Map to a Long, Loving Life Together

To defeat diabetes as quickly and effectively as possible, he's got to make the right moves . . . and that includes exercise. While he may think exercise is a nuisance, chore, or bore, just like altering his diet, exercise is an important tool in the fight to defeat diabetes. Not only will exercise help him lose weight, it will strengthen his heart, lower blood pressure, help him feel better psychologically, and reduce the risk of diabetic complications. Plus, it's great for stress reduction as well as his—and your—romantic life.

He doesn't *have* to exercise to defeat diabetes. But exercising will make it easier and quicker. Engaging in physical activity is one of the fastest ways to lower blood glucose and can reduce levels for 24 hours or more. Exercise increases insulin sensitivity, so his cells are better able to use insulin to take up glucose during and after physical activity. Plus, when muscles contract during exercise, they stimulate his cells to use glucose for energy rather than store it as fat.

Physical activity also has a big impact on psychological health, especially for type 2 diabetic males . . . like hubby. Research shows active people are less depressed than inactive people. Not only does exercise boost feel-good brain chemicals such as serotonin and endorphins, it also gives him a sense of accomplishment. Exercise also has been shown to be an effective treatment for anxiety. In other words, exercise is great for your diabetic or prediabetic partner.

Before embarking on an exercise program, it's important that he check with his doctor or health care team, especially if he is taking any diabetic medication or insulin. If he is on medication, it's important that he monitor his blood sugar correctly and avoid hypoglycemia (low blood sugar) while exercising. Otherwise, he could start feeling weak, clumsy, dizzy, or anxious. How much physical activity does he need? All adults, including your spouse, should get at least 150 minutes of moderate activity (such as brisk walking) every week. It's best to spread it out so he's exercising about 30 minutes per day five days a week. If he's out of shape or has been sedentary, he should start with 15 to 20 minutes per day and increase the amount of time he spends exercising by a few minutes each week. Doing muscle-strengthening activities (such as lifting weights or performing body weight exercises like push-ups and squats) twice a week will also provide benefits. Not only will he feel more confident and stronger, he'll build muscle mass, which will help him lose weight and reduce his blood sugar levels.

Although many people like to eat after they're done exercising, it's a good idea for your man to have a meal or snack *before* exercise for two reasons. First, he'll feel better and enjoy exercise more if he's got fuel in his system. Second, eating increases blood sugar levels, so exercising right after a meal or snack will help bring levels down quickly. If he's going to spend an hour in the gym lifting weights, he should eat a meal or snack beforehand that contains carbs. After lifting he should have a snack that contains carbs and protein (such as a banana and a cheese stick) to help him refuel and rebuild muscles.

EXCUSES: NOT ACCEPTABLE BECAUSE FAILURE IS NOT AN OPTION

Michael here. Many people hate exercising. I don't *like* to exercise. But I knew, if I was going to defeat diabetes, regain my health and vitality, and live a long, loving life with the love of my life, I really had no choice . . . and neither does your husband.

The good news is the exercises we are recommending here are really easy. Ellen is a former certified master fitness trainer (the woman has more degrees than a thermometer!), and she knows her stuff, so get your husband to listen up. These simple activities aren't designed to turn him into a barbell-eating barbarian (although barbells are very low in carbs and have tons of iron)—they're designed to lower his blood sugar.

Now let's talk about knocking down the exercise barriers, otherwise known as excuses, that many people use.

"I have no time."

Change his perception and help him prioritize. There are 10,080 minutes in a week. If he exercises just 1 percent of that time (100 minutes), it will have a big impact on helping him defeat diabetes. He can give up 1 percent of his time to save his life, right? Help him understand what's important and how much exercise will help him feel better, be healthier, and enjoy life more.

"I'm too tired."

Schedule exercise for a time of day when he feels good or the most energetic. Does he put exercise off until the end of the day and then claim he's too tired? Exercise decreases fatigue and can eliminate the stale, end-of-day, spent and exhausted feeling he finds himself in.

Numerous studies have shown that when sedentary people—both healthy adults and people with cancer, heart disease, or diabetes—start a regular, low-intensity exercise program, they experience a boost in energy levels. While researchers don't know how exercise increases energy, it's clear that exercise has a holistic, positive effect on psychological and physiological health.

"I don't feel like it."

If laziness or lack of willpower is his problem, you may need to step in because sometimes a man needs a little outside motivation. Here's one that really got *this* man's attention: remind him that exercise and sexual health are closely aligned.

"I don't like to exercise."

Join the club . . . few people do. But we're not talking about exercising to look good. We're talking about defeating diabetes, so get off your butt! There are plenty of ways to get the physical activity he needs without "exercising." Help him find activities he enjoys. It can be anything: playing Frisbee with the kids, biking, or just plain walking somewhere interesting. Even housework—vacuuming, mopping, or repairing stuff—is exercise.

DOES HE NEED TO JOIN A GYM?

Only if he wants to. Many people don't like gym environments with all those mirror-preening, muscle-bound guys grunting, "Dude, you using those 150 pound hand weights?" He doesn't need a gym to defeat diabetes. The important thing isn't *where* he exercises; it's that he increases his daily physical activity so his body can begin to process blood sugar in a more healthful manner . . . thus helping to defeat diabetes.

One benefit of gym membership is that paying a monthly fee makes him more likely to get over there and work out so the money isn't wasted. And when you're standing around a gym and everyone else is exercising, there's really only one thing to do—exercise.

KISSES, NOT CUPCAKES

He probably won't show it but inside, your newly diagnosed diabetic partner is probably upset, scared, depressed, and overwhelmed. To succeed he's going to need support and positive feedback to keep him on the defeat diabetes campaign, which can be a lonely and depressing journey on one's own. You need to help him see the big picture and keep his eye on the prize: living a long, loving life together.

Focus on improving his health and encourage him to do his part in taking care of himself. The small sacrifices—not having a second helping of pasta or that third beer, going to bed early instead of watching *The Tonight Show*, substituting a baked potato (better yet a salad) for fries—are worth making to feel better, look better, and live longer. Plus, enjoying a healthy sex life with your partner is another great benefit of defeating diabetes.

DID SOMEONE MENTION SEX?

Following our program can have a major, positive impact on your sex life. Exercise opens the arteries to the heart and increases blood flow to the penis. Research conducted at Harvard University has shown that moderate exercise (the 30-minute daily walk we're recommending) can lower his risk of and help reverse erectile dysfunction. Yep, it worked!

"Boy, did it ever."
"Is that a complaint, Ellen?"
"No, just an observation, dear."

Since Michael lost 25 pounds and his A1C dropped to 6.3, we're feeling like a couple of teenagers again. Michael has more energy and vitality, and Ellen loves her skinnier, energetic hubby.

Although 52 percent of men between the ages of 40 and 70 experience some erectile dysfunction (ED), diabetics have a significantly higher prevalence, ranging up to 75 percent. That's right, men with diabetes are two to three times more likely to have erectile dysfunction and may experience it 10 to 15 years earlier than diabetes-free men. Diabetes can damage blood vessels in the penis, making erection difficult or impossible. High blood sugar can also harm sphincter muscles, resulting in ejaculation problems. The risk of having sexual problems increases if he has poor glucose control, high cholesterol, high blood pressure, is overweight, and/or is a smoker.

Another common sexual challenge for men with diabetes is low libido. A decrease in sex drive can be triggered by several factors, including medications (especially those for depression and high blood pressure), fatigue, inactivity, and psychological issues like stress, anxiety, and depression. To make matters worse, research shows that only about half of all men with diabetes have talked to their doctor about sexual issues.

For the diabetic man, experiencing some type of sexual dysfunction or loss of desire is . . . *normal*. It's nothing to be embarrassed about and it's reversible . . . *if* he takes getting his blood sugar under control seriously. Michael did it and so can your husband.

A healthy romantic life is a great way to help him beat the diabetic blues, i.e., the depression that most men experience when they are first diagnosed. Research shows that sex helps boost mood and acts as a buffer against depression and its side effects. Yes, sex *is* nature's antidepressant. Sex is good, sex is healthy, and sex is fun.

Here are a few tips to recharge his sexual batteries and enjoy a healthy romantic life despite diabetes. As he get's healthier, these tips will become less necessary.

Stay Hydrated

This is important because dehydration can cause fatigue. When tissues are not properly hydrated, the energy needed for sexual stimulation and stamina is not generated. You've probably heard it before but it's worth repeating: try to get your husband to drink 8 to 10 glasses of water a day.

Fortify Him for Romance

Aphrodisiacs can have a powerful impact on his sex drive. There's actually real science to back it up. We wrote two books on the subject (*Food as Foreplay: Recipes for Romance, Love, and Lust,* Alexandria Press, and *Temptations: Igniting the Pleasure and Power of Aphrodisiacs,* Simon & Schuster), so we know what we're talking about. Plus, natural aphrodisiacs are a lot cheaper than Viagra, which can have unpleasant side effects.

We highly recommend having a snack prior to sex to stay energized. Make sharing a fun snack like a few chocolate-dipped strawberries part of your foreplay.

Or zinc up for fun. Found in oysters, wheat germ, and red meat, zinc is a key element of the male ejaculate. Zinc can also increase the production of libido-enhancing testosterone and help the prostate function properly. Some studies have also found it can help people with diabetes stabilize blood sugar levels. The Recommended Dietary Allowance (RDA) for men is 11 milligrams per day.

Here's another aphrodisiac we love: A study published in the *Archives of Internal Medicine* found that coffee drinking improved sex lives by increasing energy. However, don't overdo it. Stick to one cup. Too much caffeine can make him feel anxious and stressed, which will not put him in the mood.

Consider Supplements

One supplement you might suggest he take is L-arginine. Not only have several studies found that this amino acid can increase insulin sensitivity, research has shown it can also improve erections and sexual response in men. You'll find it stocked near the vitamins at the grocery store or pharmacy. Prior to taking any supplements, we recommend talking to your doctor, especially if you are on other medications.

Have a Drink

There's nothing like a glass of wine to relax him and put him in the mood. Conversely, too much alcohol can impair sexual response and reduce testosterone production.

Most people with diabetes can enjoy a moderate amount of alcohol. (No more than two drinks a day for men and one drink a day for women.) However, there are a few cautions he needs to take. He should only drink if his blood sugar is under control, and make sure he doesn't drink on an empty stomach or when blood sugar is low. Alcohol could cause hypoglycemia under those circumstances.

Plan It

Spontaneous sex is great! But between work, kids, and other responsibilities, lovemaking often doesn't happen without a plan. Will the kids be out of the house on Saturday afternoon? Can he get home from work a little early one day? A little effort goes a long way in this department. Otherwise, it's easy to let sex slide out of your schedules until it becomes an infrequent occasion rather than the regular part of your lives it should be!

Most importantly, relax and have a sense of humor about this stuff. How both of you feel about diabetes can impact your sex life. Be confident, but if something goes wrong it's no big deal. Remember, helping him defeat diabetes is the best sex strategy, and having a great sex life is a fabulous motivation to help him get and stay healthy. Just one more reason to make all the right moves!

Chapter 11

Setbacks Are Inevitable
How to Deal

Defeating diabetes will not be a smooth, downhill ride. There will be setbacks. It's completely natural. At times he will fall off the wagon and gain a pound or two back. The key is accepting setbacks as a normal part of the process . . . but not letting them become a normal part of his life again.

Here's our six-step strategy to overcome setbacks on the road to diabetes recovery.

1. Acknowledge It

Acknowledge the setback. Don't kick it under the rug. Repressed or ignored setbacks don't go away. If he doesn't bring it up, then you have to. This is especially true for emotional eating. Try to, and help him to, understand what he's going through. Is he angry with himself? Sad? Disappointed? Remember, do not judge or blame him. Reassure him that setbacks happen to everyone.

After addressing/discussing the setback, *let it go*. Don't nag or pester him. He got the message. Now move on to . . .

2. Reframe It

Reframe the setback as a learning experience. Thomas Edison failed thousands of times before inventing the light bulb. He reframed his failures by saying he had simply discovered thousands of ways that didn't work. Learning from setbacks means reframing behavior in ways that lead to success, not giving up.

Once he acknowledges the setback, see if there is something you both can learn from the experience. What led to the setback? Stress at work? An argument with you or a friend? Feeling sorry for himself? Not eating enough early in the day? (This often leads to overeating at night.) Together, figure out what he can do differently next time to avoid the setback (having healthy snacks available, lowering stress, etc.).

Next, we . . .

3. "De-catastrophize" It

While he may feel guilty and like a failure for inhaling that pint of ice cream, one meal isn't a maker or breaker on the journey to defeat diabetes. Feeling guilty will only make it worse . . . and make him more likely to overeat again to assuage his guilt, or just throw up his hands and say, "What's the use?" Help him recognize that the setback isn't as terrible as it feels. Help him accept responsibility by examining what happened and why, and how to avoid it in the future. Most of all, help him forgive himself. We all slip up . . . but winners get up. So give him a hand and help him . . .

4. Maintain a Positive Focus

We said it earlier, but it bears repeating: keep focusing on the positive. Ask him what went well in his day. Emphasize his successes, e.g., "You did great for over a week. This is just a small setback." Do something to put a smile on his face and remind him that tomorrow he'll do better, because the only way to defeat diabetes is to . . .

5. Persevere

It took years for him to develop diabetes and it's going to take time for him to defeat it. But he can do it . . . with your help. As Nelson Mandela said, "It always seems impossible until it's done." Yes, there will be some tough days, but "if you are going through hell, keep going." That was Winston Churchill, a guy who knew a thing or two about hell. Confucius said, "The man who moves a mountain begins by carrying away small stones." Get the drift?

And finally . . .

6. Accentuate the Positive

No matter what or how small his accomplishments, accentuate the positive because a lot of good things begin to happen when you fight diabetes:

✓ The energetic, pleasant way his body feels after a healthy meal will become more important than the instant fat and sugar rush of his old, deadly, diabetes-inflaming diet.

✓ His new, anti-diabetes lifestyle will also help protect him from other diseases, including arthritis, heart disease, and cancer.

✓ Children emulate adults. By taking control of his health, your mate becomes a good example and inspiration for kids and other family members. If Dad eats healthy, so will they. Get them eating right as children and they'll never need a book like this. Wouldn't that be great?

Every day you and he will be faced with numerous decisions—large and small—that can impact his health and your future together. You may feel defeated and frustrated when you see your husband engaging in behaviors that are hurting his health. In those moments you have a choice. You can do nothing, give up, get angry . . . or calmly support and guide him. You've already made a supportive choice by reading this book. Your husband is a lucky man to have a mate who loves him so much.

As the two of you work together to defeat diabetes, remember: get support for yourself, and do everything you can to optimize your own health and well-being. Let your love lead and you will make wise decisions and help your husband defeat diabetes. It's really not that hard. Michael did it, and our lives have never been better. Your husband can too.

Chapter 12

Mike and Ellen's
Diabetes-Defeating Meal Plan
(That Actually Tastes Great!)

Here it is, just like we promised, our diabetes-defeating meal plan. This is the plan Michael followed that dropped his A1C test results from 7.8 to 6.3. He reduced his total cholesterol to 198, increased his "good" HDL cholesterol to a whopping 62, and drove his triglycerides down to 110. His prostate-specific antigen (PSA, a marker for prostate cancer) was reduced to a minuscule 1.1. He lost 25 pounds and four belt notches. All this in less than a year! In other words, his change in diet changed his whole life . . . for the better.

Michael here. Being a man I hate to admit it but . . . she's right, it has changed my life. I really do feel 15 years younger. No more foot pain. No more panting up steps, sweating during short walks and easy workouts, excessive thirst, fatigue, urinating A LOT, trouble sleeping and zipping my pants, or annoying numbness and tingling. And I still get to eat the things I like . . . just not as much. Which is a small price to pay to save a life. (Especially when it's *my* life!)

Your husband can follow our plan now or face the doctor's scalpel later. Life really is at stake—don't let him throw his away for another all-you-can-eat buffet. It just isn't worth it.

Before we give you the specifics of our meal plan, Ellen wants to talk to you about a very effective, diabetes-defeating technique . . .

THE PLATE METHOD

To make portion control quick and easy, we suggest using a technique called the "plate method." A simple, effective way to help your partner lose weight and manage his blood sugar levels, the plate method will help him and you portion out the right amount of vegetables, grains, protein, dairy, and fruit at each meal.

Here's how to do it:

Start out with a 9-inch plate. Measure his from side to side to make sure it's 9 inches across! The average dinner plate used today is around 11 inches, so you may need to buy smaller plates or use a lunch plate, which typically is 9 inches. Trust us, research shows downsizing plate size is a proven weight loss tactic!

Now, let's fill that plate:

✓ *Vegetables*: Fill half of his plate with non-starchy vegetables such as lettuce, broccoli, cabbage, cauliflower, cucumbers, carrots, or celery.

✓ *Carbohydrates*: Fill one-quarter of his plate with carbs such as whole-grain bread, cooked grains (choose whole grains more often), or potatoes. The serving size for foods like grains and potatoes is approximately 1 cup, which is about the size of a fist.

✓ *Protein*: Fill the other quarter of his plate with about 4 or 5 ounces of lean protein, approximately the size of your palm. Good choices include a medium-sized fish or turkey burger, 2 eggs, a chicken thigh or breast, or a small pork chop. If you serve beans, which are a great high-fiber protein choice, consider the carbohydrate content as part of your total carbs for the entire meal, and go a little lighter on the carb quarter of the plate. Just ½ cup of beans contains approximately 20 grams of carbs, about the amount in a slice of bread or ½ cup of pasta.

✓ *Dairy*: Serve 1 cup of low-fat milk or 1 cup of yogurt on the side.

✓ *Fruit*: Serve on the side for dessert. In general, a serving is ½ cup of cut-up fruit (either fresh or unsweetened canned), 1 piece of fresh fruit (such as an apple or small banana), or 2 tablespoons dried fruit (such as raisins). Berries and melon are calorie bargains, meaning he can have 1 cup as a serving.

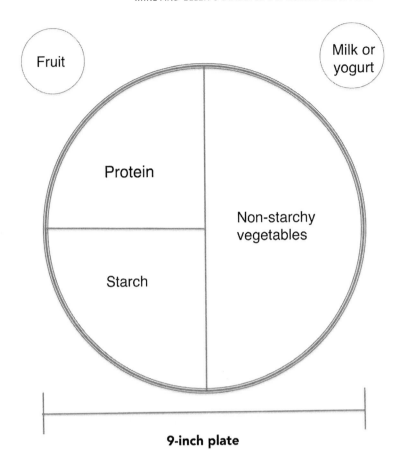

9-inch plate

ONE MORE WORD ABOUT CARBOHYDRATES (ACTUALLY 160 WORDS)

Although you do not have to count carbohydrates to reverse diabetes (Michael never did), carbs raise blood sugar more than proteins and fats, so keeping track of them can help your partner maintain healthy blood sugar levels.

Many people find counting carbs gives them a sense of control and accountability. In case you or he wants to count carbs, our meal plan includes estimated grams of carbs. The number is listed in parentheses after the food. For example, "(12)" after "1 cup low-fat milk" indicates this food contains 12 grams of carbohydrates.

We have not noted foods that may contain small amounts of carbs such as low-calorie salad dressing, nuts, or hummus. These foods are low enough in carbs that they should not have a significant impact on his blood sugar levels . . . if he does not overeat them. For more information on carb counting, refer back to chapter 6, "Scoring a Weight Loss Triple Play."

The Meal Plan

BREAKFAST

Breakfast is important! Research conducted at Tel Aviv University and published in the journal *Diabetologia* found that for people with type 2 diabetes, eating earlier in the day (when the body responds best to glucose) and less in the evening can significantly reduce blood sugar levels all day long.

Helping him eat right in the morning can be challenging. Many people don't like breakfast or feel too rushed to bother. So for your man on the go, we've put together eight healthy, tasty, filling, diabetes-defeating breakfast options. Each has about 400 calories and provides the recommended 45–60 grams of carbs he should have per meal. For meals that include low-fat milk, choose 1% or skim.

■ *Mike's Everyday Go-To Breakfast*

This is Michael's favorite quick and easy breakfast: 1 whole-wheat English muffin (30) with a teaspoon of butter, 1 hard-boiled egg, and Michael's Magic Smoothie. To make the smoothie, combine everything in the list below in a blender/mixer designed to break down fruits and vegetables into a smoothie-type drink. Now your man is ready to rock his day, every day.

½ fresh apple (8)
½ cup strawberries (7)
½ cup carrots
12 almonds
1 large handful of greens

■ *Quick, Simple, & Easy*

You can slice the banana and add it to the cereal or just eat it on the side.

> 1 cup whole-grain, high-fiber cold cereal (30)
> 1 cup low-fat milk (12)
> ½ banana (15)
> Coffee or tea with low-fat milk

■ *Stick to Your Ribs*

Make the oatmeal with the milk and sprinkle with the raisins.

> 1 cup cooked oatmeal (30)
> 1 cup low-fat milk (12)
> 2 tablespoons raisins (15)
> Coffee or tea with low-fat milk

■ *Bacon & Eggs*

Make the eggs any way he likes them. If he wants them fried, use a nonstick pan and no more than 1 teaspoon of butter or vegetable oil.

> 2 eggs
> 2 slices whole-wheat toast (30)
> 2 slices regular or turkey bacon
> 1 serving fruit (15)
> Coffee or tea with low-fat milk

■ *Yogurt, Fruit, & Granola*

Mix the berries into the yogurt and top with granola.

> ⅔ cup nonfat plain yogurt (12)
> 1 cup berries (15)
> ½ cup low-fat granola (30)
> Coffee or tea with low-fat milk

■ *PB & J*

Guys, thank me for this. She only wanted to give you 1 tablespoon of peanut butter. I love her but . . . she *is* a dietitian.

2 slices whole-grain bread (30)
2 tablespoons peanut butter
1 tablespoon jelly (13)
1 serving fruit (15)
Coffee or tea with low-fat milk

■ *Bagels & Lox*

The all-time classic made light!

½ whole-wheat bagel (30)
2 ounces smoked salmon (lox)
2 tablespoons fat-free cream cheese
1 serving fruit (15)
Coffee or tea with low-fat milk

■ *Eggs in Pita*

Add the grated cheese while scrambling the eggs, top the finished dish with the fresh salsa, and serve wrapped in the pita or tortilla.

2 eggs, scrambled
1 tablespoon grated cheese
1 6-inch whole-grain pita or 9-inch whole-wheat tortilla (30)
2 tablespoons salsa
1 serving fruit (15)
Coffee or tea with low-fat milk

LUNCH

During the week, lunch can be tricky. Temptation is a big problem at the office or work site—enticing takeout, social pressure to eat with coworkers, junk food emporiums up and down the highway. This is dangerous territory for someone trying to control diabetes. While he may plan on having just one slice of veggie pizza or a small burger and salad, his mind may quickly change when he spies the meat lover's pie or the gang is heading to the all-you-can-eat pasta buffet for lunch.

Discipline and willpower disappear when you're hungry. So how can you help him navigate the dietetically dangerous minefields that surround workplace eating? Simple . . . pack him a healthy lunch. Besides saving his health, you'll save him time, calories, and money. If he spends just $8 a day for lunch and you make a meal with $3 worth of groceries, you'll save over $1,000 a year! Just think of all the fun ways you could use that extra cash!

To make preparing a packed lunch quick and easy, follow our feng shui shopping suggestions in chapter 8 and stock up on low-calorie, flavor-packed foods. Be sure to include plenty of produce. To keep salads fresh, pack dressing separately. Make extra amounts of the main course for dinner and serve the leftovers for lunch the next day. We do this all the time with pieces of roast chicken, pork, or beef as well as soups and stir-fries.

Buy some plastic storage containers, sandwich bags, a thermos, and an insulated lunch bag to store and transport his food. If he has access to a refrigerator at work, suggest he keep a couple bottles of low-fat salad dressing there to spice up salads and as a dipping sauce for veggies.

If he doesn't have a microwave available at his work site, sandwiches are a great option . . . but skip the huge white rolls and oversized wraps. Use 2 slices of whole-grain bread, a 6-inch whole-grain pita, or a 9-inch whole-grain wrap. To keep sandwiches interesting, experiment with condiments. If he's tired of the traditional low-fat mayo or mustard sandwich, try 2 tablespoons of pesto, hummus, or avocado instead.

Here are 12 healthy, balanced lunch options he'll love.

■ The Basic Healthy Sandwich

If he likes cheese on his sandwich, that's fine—go ahead and add a slice. Don't skimp on the veggie toppings.

> 2 slices whole-wheat bread, 1 6-inch whole-grain pita
>   pocket, or 1 9-inch wrap (30)
> 4 ounces lean roast beef, ham, turkey, or soy "meat"
> 2 tablespoons low-fat mayo, mustard, or hummus

Lettuce, tomato, sprouts, bell peppers, spinach,
   or grated carrots
1 cup low-fat milk or 6 ounces yogurt (12)
1 serving fruit (15)

■ Mediterranean Chicken Wrap

Wraps are increasingly popular offerings at grocery and convenience store delis, but they're just as easy to make as any sandwich. For our take on the classic wrap, combine the chicken, feta cheese, red peppers, and olives. Spread the greens over the tortilla, top with chicken/feta mixture, and roll up tightly.

4 ounces grilled, baked, or sautéed chicken breast, shredded
1 ounce crumbled feta cheese
1 9-inch whole-grain tortilla (30)
2 tablespoons roasted red peppers, chopped
2 tablespoons black olives, chopped
Small handful baby spinach, lettuce, or arugula
1 cup low-fat milk or 6 ounces yogurt (12)
1 serving fruit (15)

■ The Bacon Lover's BLT

No, he doesn't have to give up his lunchtime bacon, lettuce, and tomato! We've hacked the BLT and made it diabetic-friendly. By replacing regular, high-fat bacon with slices of Canadian bacon, he saves 125 calories and 25 grams of fat without having to sacrifice flavor. Try it. He'll like it!

4 slices (about 4 ounces) Canadian bacon
1 medium whole-grain French roll (30)
1 tablespoon low-fat mayo
Sliced tomato
Lettuce
½ cup baby carrot sticks
¾ ounce baked potato chips, about 10 to 12 chips (15)
1 piece fruit (15)

There are plenty of other healthy, no-microwave options than just sandwiches. He can take soups, leftover stews, and chili hot from home in a thermos. This is great for guys who are microwave challenged, like the fool who puts a whole can of chicken soup (still in the can) in the office microwave . . . until it explodes! Yes, that person is someone's husband. Yours?

Here are a few more "no microwave necessary" lunches.

■ *Salmon Salad*

When you combine the salmon and mayo, add chopped onion or capers for extra flavor if he likes, and feel free to substitute canned tuna packed in water for the salmon. The crackers are for the salmon salad and the hummus is a dip for the veggies.

4 ounces canned salmon packed in water
1 tablespoon low-fat mayo
20 small whole-grain crackers or snack chips (30)
1 cup broccoli florets or baby carrots
2 tablespoons hummus or low-fat salad dressing
1 serving fruit (15)
1 cup low-fat milk (12)

■ *Manly Salad*

Top the greens with the meat, egg, and cheese for a hearty lunchtime salad.

2 cups mixed dark greens
2 ounces cooked chicken breast or sliced ham, turkey,
   or lean beef
1 hard-boiled egg
1 ounce cheese, shredded or cubed
2 tablespoons light salad dressing of his choice
1 medium whole-grain roll or 2 slices whole-wheat bread (30)
1 cup low-fat milk (12)
1 piece fruit (15)

If he has a microwave available at work, his healthy lunch options are plentiful.

■ *Chili & Chips*

Heat the chili in the microwave at work, or heat it at home and bring to work in a thermos. Top with his choice of shredded cheddar cheese or the yogurt. If you choose the potato as the side, have him microwave it at work to cook it.

> 1 cup chili
> 2 tablespoons cheddar cheese or nonfat yogurt
> Salsa, as much as he likes
> 1½ ounces baked corn chips or 1 medium-sized
>   baked potato (30)
> Salad with 2 tablespoons low-fat dressing
> 1 serving fruit (15)
> 1 cup low-fat milk (12)

■ *Cupa Soup*

Short on time? Feel free to substitute healthy canned soup. (Remember, read the label!)

> 1 cup bean, lentil, split pea, or chicken soup (15)
> 12 whole-grain crackers or a small whole-wheat roll (15)
> Salad with 2 tablespoons low-fat dressing
> 6 ounces low-fat yogurt (12)
> 1 serving fruit (15)

■ *Pasta Lunch*

Prepare the pasta and meatballs at home the night before. For the sauce, skip the high-fat Alfredo sauce and instead choose any number of jarred marinara sauces. Heat in the microwave.

> 1 cup whole-wheat pasta (30)
> ½ cup marinara sauce
> 3 ounces cooked turkey meatballs
> Salad with 2 tablespoons low-fat dressing
> 1 cup low-fat milk (12)
> 1 serving fruit (15)

■ *Refried Beans & Chips*

You'll usually find cans of refried beans stocked with the canned vegetables or in the Mexican specialty section of your supermarket. Sprinkle with the cheese and heat in the microwave.

> ½ cup low-fat refried beans (15)
> 1 ounce shredded cheese
> 1½ ounces baked corn chips (30)
> Salsa, as much as he likes
> Salad with 2 tablespoons low-fat dressing
> 1 serving fruit (15)

■ *Veggie Burger*

Veggie burgers generally come frozen and can be heated in the microwave. It doesn't get easier than that.

> 1 veggie burger (15)
> Condiment of his choice
> 1 slice of cheese (about 1 ounce)
> 1 medium whole-wheat roll or 2 slices whole-wheat bead (30)
> Low-fat coleslaw or salad with 2 tablespoons low-fat dressing
> 1 serving fruit (15)

For a fun weekend lunch at home, have him try these:

■ *Pizza Muffin*

Split the muffin and top each half with the sauce, cheese, and meat. Broil in toaster oven until the cheese melts.

> 1 small whole-wheat English muffin (30)
> ¼ to ½ cup tomato or pizza sauce
> ¼ cup shredded part-skim mozzarella cheese
> 2 ounces turkey sausage or turkey pepperoni
> Salad with 2 tablespoon low-fat dressing
> 1 cup low-fat milk (12)
> 1 serving fruit (15)

■ *Tuna Melt*

When you mix the tuna with the mayo, add chopped or minced pickle, capers, celery, or whatever produce-based flavor enhancer he likes. Top the toasted English muffin or roll with the tuna and cheese and broil until the cheese melts.

> 1 small whole-wheat English muffin or split
>   whole-grain roll (30)
> 4 ounces tuna mixed with 1½ teaspoons light mayo
> 1 ounce cheese of choice
> 1 serving fruit (15)
> 1 cup low-fat milk (15)

DINNER

Most of us are accustomed to enjoying a big dinner, especially after a hard day at work. The key to satisfying him—and defeating diabetes—is to make it big *and* healthy! (The secret to making it big is sneaking in lots of veggies.)

We know you work hard too, so we've designed two weeks' worth of quick, healthy meal options he'll love, plus three fun ones for Saturday night. And we'll tell you exactly how to make each one of our delicious, diabetes-defeating entrées. If your kitchen is stocked as we outlined in chapter 8, you can whip up these healthy meals quickly and easily. For meals calling for a side salad, mix it up—tossed lettuce salad one night, spinach salad the next, mixed greens the next.

■ *Baked Fish*

Here is a super simple way to prepare a tasty, healthy fish dinner.

> 4–5 ounces Baked Fish
> 1 cup steamed or boiled green beans
> 1 6-ounce baked potato (30) with
> 2 tablespoons fat-free sour cream or yogurt or 1 teaspoon butter
> 1 small whole-grain dinner roll (15)
> ½ cup low-fat frozen yogurt (15)

To prepare the fish (serves 3–4):

INGREDIENTS

1 pound white fish such as haddock, cod, or tilapia
Salt and pepper, to taste
1 tablespoon butter, melted
1 teaspoon lemon juice
2 cloves garlic, minced
1½ teaspoons fresh herbs such as parsley, thyme, tarragon,
   or basil, minced, or ½ teaspoon dried herbs

DIRECTIONS

1. Preheat oven to 350° F. Lightly grease a baking dish with non-stick cooking spray.
2. Rinse and pat fish dry with a paper towel. Arrange fish in prepared dish and sprinkle with salt and pepper.
3. In a medium bowl, combine melted butter, lemon juice, minced garlic, and herbs. Brush mixture evenly over fish.
4. Bake until fish is opaque and flakes easily, about 25–30 minutes.

■ Stir-Fried Shrimp, Chicken, Pork, or Tofu with Vegetables

Our simple take on the classic Asian dish. Yes, occasionally it's okay to enjoy white rice. This stir-fry is fast, filling, and so much healthier than takeout!

1 serving Stir-Fried Shrimp, Chicken, Pork, or Tofu
   with Vegetables
1 cup cooked white rice (45)
2 tablespoons crushed peanuts for garnish
1 cup whole strawberries (13)

To prepare the stir-fry (serves 4):

INGREDIENTS

1 cup chicken broth
2 tablespoons soy sauce
1 tablespoon sugar
1 tablespoon rice or white vinegar

    1 teaspoon cornstarch

    2 tablespoons vegetable oil

    1 pound mixed vegetables (such as onions, carrots, peppers, and broccoli) cut into bite-sized pieces (or use frozen Asian mixed vegetables)

    1 tablespoon garlic, ginger, and/or shallots, chopped

    1 pound chicken, beef, pork, shrimp, or tofu, cut into bite-sized pieces

DIRECTIONS

1. Mix sauce ingredients—chicken broth, soy sauce, sugar, vinegar, and cornstarch—in a medium bowl and set aside.
2. Heat 1 tablespoon vegetable oil in a large nonstick sauté pan over high heat. Add vegetables and cook, stirring occasionally, until tender, about 6–8 minutes. Add garlic, ginger, and/or shallots and cook for 1 more minute. Pour into a bowl, cover to keep warm, and set aside.
3. Wipe pan clean with a paper towel. (Careful, it's still hot.) Add remaining tablespoon of oil and heat on high. When oil is hot add shrimp, chicken, beef, pork, or tofu and stir-fry until meat or poultry is cooked through, shrimp is opaque, or tofu is nicely browned. (If you choose shrimp, remember—it cooks quickly. It should only take about 3 to 5 minutes.)
4. Pour the reserved vegetables and sauce back into the pan. Stir to combine. Lower heat to medium and cook until sauce thickens, about 1–2 minutes.
5. Serve over rice, topped with peanuts.

■ *Roast Whole Chicken*

A quick, simple, and tasty way to cook chicken. If he sneaks a little more of the chicken onto his plate, that's okay. Use leftovers for lunches and snacks.

    1 4 to 6-ounce piece of chicken

    1 6-ounce baked potato (30) with

    1 teaspoon butter or 2 tablespoons fat-free sour cream

    1 cup steamed or boiled broccoli topped with lemon juice

1 serving fruit (15)
1 cup low-fat milk (12)

To prepare the chicken (serves 4–5):

INGREDIENTS
1 teaspoon dried mixed herbs (such as Italian herbs
or herbes de Provence)
2 cloves garlic, minced
2 tablespoons olive oil
1 whole chicken (4–5 pounds), butterflied (e.g., take out the
back with poultry shears) or split
Salt and pepper, to taste

DIRECTIONS
1. Preheat oven to 500° F.
2. In a small bowl, mix the herbs, garlic, and 1 tablespoon olive oil
   with ½ teaspoon salt and ¼ teaspoon pepper.
3. Place chicken in large roasting or jelly roll pan. Loosen breast
   and thigh skin and rub herb-garlic mixture underneath.
4. Rub skin with remaining tablespoon of olive oil and sprinkle
   with salt and pepper to taste.
5. Roast on lower-middle rack of oven until chicken is nicely
   brown, juices are clear, and internal temperature is 165° F, about
   45 minutes to 1 hour.

■ *Maple Salmon*

Don't worry about the maple syrup in the main dish. The recipe
calls for just a small amount in the marinade. He won't be consuming too much sugar.

4–6 ounces Maple Salmon (14)
⅔ cup brown rice (30)
Salad with 2 tablespoons low-fat dressing
1 cup berries (15)

To prepare the salmon (serves 3–4):

INGREDIENTS

¼ cup maple syrup
2 tablespoons soy sauce
2 cloves garlic, minced
1 pound salmon filet

DIRECTIONS

1. In a medium bowl, combine maple syrup, soy sauce, and garlic.
2. Place salmon in a shallow baking dish. Pour maple syrup, soy sauce, and garlic mixture over salmon, cover dish, and marinate for 30 minutes in the refrigerator, turning once.
3. Preheat oven to 400° F.
4. Roast salmon in preheated oven, uncovered, until fish is opaque and flakes easily with a fork, about 20 minutes.

■ *Veggie Burrito*

These burritos freeze really well and are great to take to work for lunch. Plus they're super high in fiber! You can substitute any reduced-fat cheese he prefers for the Mexican blend.

1 Veggie Burrito (35)
½ cup salsa
Salad with 2 tablespoons low-fat dressing
1 serving fruit (15)
½ cup frozen yogurt (15)

To prepare the burritos (serves 6):

INGREDIENTS

1 can (16 ounces) vegetarian low-fat or fat-free refried beans
1 1-pound bag frozen mixed vegetables
1 cup cooked brown rice
1 teaspoon garlic powder
1 cup salsa
4 ounces (about 1 cup) shredded reduced-fat Mexican cheese blend
6 8-inch whole-wheat flour tortillas

DIRECTIONS

1. Preheat oven to 350° F. Coat a baking dish with nonstick cooking spray.
2. In a large bowl combine refried beans, vegetables, rice, garlic powder, ½ cup salsa, and ½ cup cheese.
3. Put 1 tortilla on a plate. Spread about 1 cup of the bean, rice, vegetable, and cheese mixture in the tortilla, roll up, and place in prepared pan. Repeat with remaining tortillas.
4. Spread remaining ½ cup salsa over the wrapped tortillas and top with remaining ½ cup cheese. Bake in preheated oven until cheese is browned, about 30 minutes.

■ Chicken, Shrimp, or Beef Fajitas

A quick, healthy midweek meal that's still lots of fun. Use more of the chili powder if he likes spicy food and less if he doesn't.

4 ounces fajita-style chicken, shrimp, or beef
2 6-inch whole-wheat tortillas (30)
Salsa
1 serving fruit (15)
1 cup low-fat milk (12)

To prepare the fajitas (serves 4):

INGREDIENTS

2 teaspoons vegetable oil
1 medium onion, sliced
2 bell peppers (any color you like), seeded and cut into
    ¼-inch-wide strips
1 pound boneless, skinless chicken breast or lean beef cut
    into 2-inch strips against the grain, or pealed and deveined
    shrimp
½ teaspoon garlic powder
1½ teaspoons ground cumin
1–2 teaspoons chili powder
Salt and pepper, to taste
8 6-inch whole-wheat tortillas

DIRECTIONS

1. Wrap tortillas in tinfoil and warm in 250° F oven.
2. Heat 1 teaspoon vegetable oil in a large nonstick skillet over medium-high heat. When skillet is hot, add onions and bell peppers. Cook until vegetables are soft, about 6–8 minutes. Remove vegetables from pan and cover to keep warm.
3. Heat remaining teaspoon of vegetable oil in skillet over medium-high heat. When skillet is hot add chicken, beef, or shrimp. Cook, stirring frequently, until chicken or beef is no longer pink or until shrimp is opaque, about 6–10 minutes for beef or chicken and 3–5 minutes for shrimp.
4. Add garlic, cumin, and chili powder, stir, and cook for another 30 seconds. Add cooked vegetables, then season with salt and pepper to taste. Serve in warmed tortillas topped with favorite garnishes such as lime juice (seriously, it's delicious), nonfat sour cream, or salsa.

■ Turkey Chili

This spicy, hearty chili is terrific with chips, on a baked potato, or over pasta. If you're short on time, substitute canned low-fat turkey chili.

> 1 cup Turkey Chili (7)
> 1 ounce cheddar cheese, grated
> ½ cup salsa
> 1½ ounces baked corn chips or 1 6-ounce baked potato (30)
> Salad with 2 tablespoons low-fat dressing
> 1 serving fruit (15)

To prepare the chili (serves 8):

INGREDIENTS

> 1 tablespoon vegetable oil
> 1 pound ground turkey
> 1 large onion, chopped
> 2 carrots, chopped
> 1 bell pepper (any color), seeded and chopped
> 1½ cups tomato sauce

1½ cups salsa

1 can (14½ ounces) beans such as kidney or black,
   drained and rinsed

1 tablespoon chili powder

½ teaspoon dried oregano

DIRECTIONS

1. Heat vegetable oil in a large pot over medium-high heat. Add turkey and cook, breaking up pieces with a spatula, until no longer pink, about 6–8 minutes.
2. Add onion, carrots, and bell pepper and cook until vegetables are soft, about 6–8 minutes.
3. Add tomato sauce, salsa, beans, chili powder, and oregano. Bring to a simmer, and cook for 15 minutes, stirring occasionally. Serve.

■ *Classic Mac & Cheese*

Not from a box! So good you might need a pitchfork to hold hubby off from taking seconds, thirds . . .

1 main course serving Classic Mac & Cheese (40)

1 cup tomato soup

Salad topped with 2 tablespoons low-fat dressing

1 cup low-fat milk (12)

To prepare the mac and cheese (serves 4 as main course, 8 as a side dish):

INGREDIENTS

½ pound whole-wheat pasta such as rotini or elbows

2 cups broccoli florets

2 eggs

1 can (12 ounces) evaporated low-fat milk

¼ teaspoon hot pepper sauce

1 teaspoon Dijon mustard

1 cup reduced-fat cheddar cheese, shredded

4 ounces Canadian bacon, cut into bite-sized pieces

⅓ cup seasoned bread crumbs

⅓ cup grated Parmesan cheese
Salt and pepper, to taste

DIRECTIONS
1. Preheat oven to 400° F. Coat a 9 x 9–inch or similar size baking dish with nonstick cooking spray and set aside.
2. Bring a large pot of salted water to a boil. Add pasta. When pasta is about 1 minute from being done, add broccoli. Continue cooking for another minute and drain pasta and broccoli.
3. Combine eggs, evaporated milk, mustard, hot pepper sauce, cheese and Canadian bacon. Toss mixture with pasta and broccoli. Season with salt and pepper to taste.
4. Pour the mixture into prepared pan. Top with bread crumbs and Parmesan cheese. Bake in preheated oven until golden brown, about 20 minutes.

■ Entrée Salad

The perfect meal for hot summer nights or when you just don't feel like cooking.

¼ cup cannellini or garbanzo beans (7)
3 ounces cooked, chopped chicken breast or lean steak
1 ounce cheese or 1 hard-boiled egg
2 tablespoons low-fat salad dressing
1 medium whole-grain roll or 1 cup whole-grain pasta (30)
1 serving fruit (15)

To prepare the salad (serves 4):

INGREDIENTS
4 cups washed salad greens
Chopped or sliced vegetables such as cucumbers, broccoli, peppers, carrots, olives, or tomatoes
1 cup cannellini or garbanzo beans
12 ounces cooked, cubed chicken breast or lean steak strips
4 ounces reduced-fat shredded cheese or 4 sliced hard-boiled eggs

DIRECTIONS
1. Combine salad greens and vegetables in a large bowl.
2. Top greens with beans and either chicken or steak. Top off with either eggs or cheese.

■ Burger Meister

Keep frozen salmon and turkey burgers on hand for a fun, quick, and healthy meal. Top his burger with as much lettuce, tomato, pickles, or red onion as he likes, in whatever ratio he likes. Serve with our Oven Fries . . . up next. Follow package instructions to prepare burger.

> 1 4-ounce cooked salmon or turkey burger
> Lettuce, tomato, pickles, or red onion
> 1 medium whole-wheat bun (30)
> 1 serving Oven Fries (30)
> Salad with 2 tablespoons low-fat dressing

■ Oven Fries

So good he won't miss those high-calorie, deep-fried, French diabetic bombshells. (We're not talking about Brigitte Bardot.)

To prepare the fries (serves 4):

INGREDIENTS
> 3 medium baking potatoes cut into ¼-inch-wide sticks
> 2 tablespoons olive oil
> Salt and pepper, to taste

DIRECTIONS
1. Preheat oven to 425° F. Coat a jelly roll pan with cooking spray.
2. In a large bowl, toss potatoes with oil and ½ teaspoon salt.
3. Spread potatoes in prepared pan. Bake, turning once, until golden and crisp, about 35 minutes. When fries are almost ready, cook your burger. Season with salt and pepper to taste.

■ *Super Sausage Supper*

A super easy supper that's packed with filling fiber. Leftovers are great warm or cold the next day for lunch.

1 serving Super Sausage Supper (15)
1 cup whole-grain pasta (30)
1 serving fruit (15)

To prepare the sausage (serves 4):

INGREDIENTS

1 teaspoon olive oil
1 large onion, chopped
1 bell pepper, chopped
2 cups broccoli florets
¼ cup black, pitted olives, drained
½ teaspoon garlic powder
½ teaspoon Italian herbs
1 can (14½ ounce) white beans (cannellini or other)
Salt and pepper, to taste
4 fully cooked chicken sausages
¼ cup grated Parmesan cheese

DIRECTIONS

1. Preheat oven to 350° F. Cook chicken sausages in oven until browned and heated through, about 10 minutes.
2. Heat olive oil in a large nonstick sauté pan over medium-high heat. Add onions and peppers and sauté until tender, about 6–8 minutes. Add broccoli and cook until bright green. Stir in olives, garlic powder, Italian herbs, and beans. Cook until heated through, about 2 minutes. Add salt and pepper to taste.
3. Preheat broiler.
4. Place sausages in pan with vegetables and beans. Top with cheese. Broil until cheese is browned, about 3–5 minutes. (Don't use a pan with a plastic handle for this recipe—it will melt under the broiler!)
5. Serve over cooked whole-grain pasta.

■ *Veggie Frittata*

"Frittata" is just a fancy way of saying "unfolded omelet." Feel free to substitute different vegetables such as broccoli or zucchini for the bell pepper and spinach in the main dish.

> 1 serving Veggie Frittata
> 2 slices whole-grain bread, 1 medium whole-grain roll,
>   or 1 whole-wheat English muffin (30)
> 1 serving fruit (15)
> ½ cup frozen yogurt (15)

To prepare the frittata (serves 4):

INGREDIENTS

> 1½ teaspoons olive oil
> 1 medium onion, chopped
> 1 red bell pepper, seeded and chopped
> 2 cups (packed) baby spinach leaves
> 8 large eggs
> ½ teaspoon dried mixed herbs
> Salt and pepper, to taste
> ¼ cup (1 ounce) grated Parmesan or Asiago cheese

DIRECTIONS

1. Heat olive oil in large nonstick skillet over medium-high heat. Add onion and bell pepper. Sauté until vegetables are tender, about 6–8 minutes. Add spinach and stir until wilted, about 1 minute.
2. Wisk eggs with herbs, salt, and pepper in medium bowl to blend. Pour egg mixture over hot vegetables in skillet. Stir gently to combine. Reduce heat to medium-low. Cook without stirring until eggs are set on bottom, about 5 minutes.
3. Preheat boiler. Sprinkle cheese over eggs, then broil until cheese melts, about 2 minutes. (Remember, don't use a pan with a plastic handle—it will melt under the broiler!)
4. Cut into wedges and enjoy.

■ *Michael's Minestrone Soup*

Perfect for cool nights, this soup will fill hubby up and warm his heart.

> 2 cups Michael's Minestrone (30)
> 1 small dinner roll or ¾ ounce whole-grain crackers (15)
> Salad with 2 tablespoons low-fat dressing
> 1 serving fruit (15)

To prepare the soup (serves 6):

INGREDIENTS
> 1 tablespoon olive oil
> 1 onion, chopped
> 2 carrots, chopped
> 2 celery stalks, chopped
> 2 cloves garlic, minced
> 2 teaspoons dried herbs such as oregano, basil, or thyme
> 1 can (14½ ounces) diced tomatoes
> 6 cups chicken stock
> 1 can (14½ ounces) white or kidney beans, rinsed and drained
> 4 ounces uncooked whole-wheat pasta (about 1 cup)
> Salt and pepper, to taste

DIRECTIONS
1. Heat oil in a heavy-bottomed stockpot or Dutch oven over medium-high heat.
2. Add onion, carrot, celery, and garlic. Cook, stirring frequently, until vegetables are soft, about 6–8 minutes.
3. Stir in herbs, tomatoes, and stock. Bring soup to a boil, reduce heat, and simmer uncovered for 10 minutes.
4. Add beans and pasta. Bring back to a simmer and cook until pasta is tender, about 10–13 minutes. Add salt and pepper to taste.

■ *Herb-Roasted Vegetables*

This dish is extremely easy to prepare and wonderful served hot or cold. Feel free to use the vegetables he likes best; just remember that starchy vegetables such as potatoes and squash count as carbs.

> 1 serving Herb-Roasted Vegetables (25)
> 4 ounces cheese, cold chicken, or sliced steak
> 1 cup low-fat milk (12)
> ½ cup frozen yogurt (15)

To prepare the vegetables (serves 4):

INGREDIENTS

> 2 large onions, cut into wedges
> 2 sweet potatoes, cut into bite-size pieces
> 2 white potatoes, cut into bite-size pieces
> 1 small butternut squash, cut into bite-size pieces
> ½ cup baby carrots
> ½ head cauliflower, cut into florets
> 1 head of garlic, separated into cloves
> ¼ cup olive oil
> 2 teaspoons dried mixed herbs
> Salt and pepper, to taste
> 2 tablespoons balsamic vinegar

DIRECTIONS

1. Preheat oven to 425° F.
2. In a large bowl combine all vegetables. Toss with olive oil, herbs, and salt and pepper to taste.
3. Spread vegetables into large roasting pan or two smaller roasting pans.
4. Roast for 35 to 40 minutes in preheated oven, stirring every 10–15 minutes, until vegetables are tender and browned. Toss with balsamic vinegar and serve.

SATURDAY NIGHT FLAVOR RECIPES

It's Saturday night and time for fun! He's been good all week so reward him with one of our favorite fun (but still healthy) recipes. Let flavor rule . . . and fuel his Saturday Night Fever.

■ *Saturday Night Steak*

This elegant little meal features sliced sirloin steak with a wine reduction. The recipe leaves room for leftovers, but will there be any?

> 4–8 ounces Saturday Night Steak, sliced
> 1 6-ounce baked potato (30)
> 1 small whole-grain roll (15)
> 1 teaspoon butter
> Salad with 2 tablespoons low-fat dressing
> Small brownie (15)

To prepare the steak (serves 4 to 6):

INGREDIENTS

> 1 1½–2 pound sirloin steak at least 1-inch thick
> Salt and pepper, to taste
> 2 cloves garlic, minced
> 1 tablespoon balsamic vinegar
> ¼ cup dry sherry
> 2 tablespoon soy sauce
> 1 tablespoon honey

DIRECTIONS

1. Sprinkle both sides of steaks with salt and pepper to taste, then press the salt and pepper into the meat with your fingers.
2. Heat a skillet over medium-high. (It should be large enough so the steak will not touch the sides.) Test the pan with a piece of beef fat from the steak. If the fat does not sizzle immediately, the pan is not hot enough yet. When fully heated, add steak to pan and cook approximately 4–5 minutes per side or until

desired degree of doneness. Remove steak from pan and cover with foil to keep warm. The steak will continue to cook wrapped in foil, so take it off a bit before it reaches your favorite stage of doneness.

3. Place pan back on stove and heat over medium-high. Add garlic to pan and sauté for 30 seconds, scraping up any browned bits. Add balsamic vinegar and sherry to pan and bring to a boil. Cook for 30 seconds. Add soy sauce and honey, bring to a boil, and cook for 1 minute, stirring occasionally. Serve sauce over slices of steak or on the side for dipping.

■ *Veggie Pizza*

Feel free to substitute different vegetables and cheeses when creating your pizza.

1 serving Veggie Pizza (33)
Salad with 2 tablespoons low-fat dressing
1 serving fruit (15)
½ cup frozen yogurt (15)

To prepare the pizza (serves 4):

INGREDIENTS

1 12-inch whole-wheat thin pizza crust
1 cup pizza sauce
1 cup fresh broccoli, chopped
1 cup marinated artichoke hearts, drained and chopped
1 cup mushrooms, sliced
2 cups low-fat mozzarella cheese, shredded

DIRECTIONS

1. Preheat oven to 450°F.
2. Spread sauce on crust, leaving 1-inch border. Top with veggies and cheese. Bake until cheese is melted and crust is golden brown, about 10–12 minutes.

■ *Oven-Fried Chicken Wings*

Michael's favorite and much healthier than what Fast Food Freddy grabs at The Chicken Shack Fry Stand! Serve him four whole wings with Buffalo hot sauce and a side of celery.

>1 serving Oven-Fried Chicken Wings (15)
>1 serving Oven Fries (30)
>Cut-up veggies with 2 tablespoons low-fat salad dressing
>1 serving fruit (15)

To prepare the wings (serves 4):

INGREDIENTS

>1 cup low-fat milk
>2 tablespoons lemon juice
>½ teaspoon garlic powder
>Dash hot pepper sauce
>Salt and pepper, to taste
>2 pounds chicken wings
>½ cup seasoned Italian bread crumbs
>½ cup cornmeal

DIRECTIONS

1. Combine milk, lemon juice, garlic, hot sauce, salt, and pepper in a sealable plastic bag or large bowl. Add wings, seal bag or cover bowl, and let marinate in the refrigerator for 2–4 hours.
2. Heat oven to 425° F. Lightly grease a large jelly roll or roasting pan with nonstick cooking spray.
3. Combine breadcrumbs, cornmeal, and a little more salt and pepper to taste in a clean bag. Remove chicken from marinade. Add half the wings to bread crumb/cornmeal mixture, seal bag, and shake to coat wings. Place coated wings, skin side up, in prepared pan. Repeat with remaining wings.
4. Bake in preheated oven until wings are golden and tender, about 35–40 minutes.

Appendix

Helpful Resources

Ellen and Michael have developed the following websites to guide you on your weight loss journey and support health and well-being, increase your longevity, and yes, defeat diabetes!

SmashYourScale.com
WellCouples.com
DrEllenAlbertson.com

As you embark on your campaign to defeat diabetes, you will undoubtedly come across dozens of books, magazine articles, and websites loaded with information, anecdotes, and advice. It can be overwhelming! We've simplified things for you greatly by offering this quick list of credible, no-nonsense resources for the latest information on diabetes, nutrition and wellness.

American Diabetes Association
www.diabetes.org
The American Diabetes Association is a great place to go for information on diabetes basics, living with diabetes, the latest research, and more.

Academy of Nutrition and Dietetics
www.eatright.org
The Academy of Nutrition and Dietetics is the world's largest organization of food and nutrition professionals. On the site you'll find hundreds of articles on food, nutrition, health and fitness as well as instructional videos and healthy, delicious recipes from registered dietitians.

Fast Food Nutrition
www.fastfoodnutrition.org
This handy, easy-to-use website, contains nutrition facts for thousands of menu items from the most popular fast food eateries. Be sure to utilize the Meal Nutrition Facts Calculator before you hit the drive-thru!

American Heart Association
www.heart.org
Because diabetes and heart disease are so closely linked, you should familiarize yourself with the information and resources available through this website. The association was founded by six cardiologists in 1924 and has since grown into the preeminent nonprofit organization for all things related to heart health.

Office of Disease Prevention and Health Promotion
www.health.gov
This division of the US Department of Health and Human Services is a great resource for general information on living a fit, healthy life. It is where you will find the latest American Dietary Guidelines.

Mayo Clinic
www.mayoclinic.org
No, it's not a school for how to make deli sandwiches. Founded in Rochester, Minnesota in 1889, today the Mayo Clinic is one of the most respected medical institutions in the world. The Mayo Clinic is an excellent resource for unbiased medical information.